OFFICE OF POPULATION CENSUSES AND SURVEYS
SOCIAL SURVEY DIVISION

Children's dental health in the United Kingdom 1983

A survey carried out by the Social Survey Division of OPCS, on behalf of the United Kingdom health departments, in collaboration with the Dental Schools of the Universities of Birmingham and Newcastle

**Jean E Todd
Tricia Dodd**

London: Her Majesty's Stationery Office

ISBN 0 11 691136 0

Acknowledgements

This study was carried out in the first quarter of 1983 by OPCS in collaboration with the dental schools at the Universities of Birmingham and Newcastle, and we would like to thank all of the individuals in those organisations who helped with the successful launch and completion of the study.

We would also like to thank the regional organisers and the dentists and their recorders who went through the training course and subsequently carried out 20,000 dental examinations.

These examinations took place in schools, and we would like to thank the Local Education Authorities and the sampled schools for their help and co-operation in administering the study.

We would also like to say thank you to the 20,000 children who agreed to be examined for the survey, and we would especially like to thank the children who volunteered to help us in the training course, they were examined not once but innumerable times.

We also wrote to the parents of a sample of the children and asked them to fill in a questionnaire about the child's dental background, and we would like to thank all those who completed it and returned it to us; 95% of parents who were sent a questionnaire co-operated in this way including one who mislaid it at the time but returned it in October 1984, just before we went to print. We could not at that stage include this last questionnaire in the survey findings, but by mentioning it here we have managed to include it in the report.

To all those who took part in any way we express our thanks and appreciation for making the survey of children's dental health possible.

Contents

Notes on the tables

The varying positions of percentage signs in the tables denote the presentation of different types of information. Where the percentage sign is at the head of a column the whole distribution is presented. (Figures may not add to 100 however due to rounding.) A percentage sign at the side of an individual figure signifies that this proportion of children had the attribute being discussed and that the complementary proportion (not shown in the table) did not.

Where a base number is less than 30, statistics have not been given and this is indicated by an asterisk. A dash in a table represents a proportion of less than 0.5% or a mean of less than 0.05 or a zero value.

1 Introduction

1.1 Background to the survey

In 1973 the first national study of children's dental health[1] was carried out by Social Survey Division of the Office of Population Censuses and Surveys (OPCS) in collaboration with the Department of Dental Health, University of Birmingham on behalf of the Department of Health and Social Security (DHSS). The survey covered children in maintained schools in England and Wales aged five to fifteen. When that survey was planned, it was envisaged that future surveys would be carried out to measure changes in dental health from the baseline established in 1973, and, ten years after the original survey, OPCS was again commissioned to carry out a survey of children's dental health in collaboration with the dental schools at the Universities of Birmingham and Newcastle. However, in 1983, the survey was commissioned not only by the DHSS in conjunction with the Welsh Office for England and Wales but also by the Scottish Home and Health Department and the Department of Health and Social Services in Northern Ireland, so that, for the first time, information on children's dental health in the United Kingdom was collected. The sample for the survey was designed so that separate analyses could be carried out for England, Wales, Scotland and Northern Ireland, which entailed the selection of a proportionately larger sample of children in Wales, Scotland and Northern Ireland, compared with England.

As in 1973, the survey involved a dental examination (carried out in school) of all the selected children, and the collection of background information from the parents of a sample of the selected children. The development of the criteria used in the dental examination and the training of the dental team to carry out this examination was undertaken jointly by the Department of Dental Health at the University of Birmingham Dental School and the Department of Child Dental Health at the University of Newcastle Dental School.

The proposals for the survey and for the examination criteria were discussed with and agreed by a dental steering committee comprising representatives from the commissioning departments, the university dental schools, the community dental service and professional organisations.

The survey was piloted in the Autumn of 1982 and the main fieldwork took place in January and February 1983.

1.2 The sample

The sample for the survey covered all children in non-private schools in the United Kingdom aged between five and fifteen inclusively. The sampling of the children in England, Wales and Scotland was the responsibility of OPCS while the Department of Health and Social Services was responsible for the sampling of the children in Northern Ireland.

The first stage of the sampling was to achieve a nationally representative sample of non-private schools. This sampling was, for administrative reasons, carried out slightly differently for England and Wales and for Scotland and Northern Ireland.

In England and Wales, the Department of Education and Science (DES) keep on record information regarding all maintained schools, including their size, age groups of the children etc but not their addresses. The addresses of all secondary maintained schools appear in the Education Year Book. The addresses of primary schools do not appear in any official lists but are kept centrally at the Department of Education and Science. There are over 23,000 primary schools in England and Wales and it would have been extremely time consuming to locate each one before the initial sample was drawn. It was therefore decided to base the sample, initially, on secondary schools because their locations were readily available.

All secondary schools in England and Wales were allocated to their relevant local authority district or London Borough and the total number of school children aged eleven to fifteen was calculated for each district. Districts were then selected with probability proportional to the number of secondary school children in them. In England, 60 selections were taken and in Wales, 20 selections were taken.

The secondary schools within each of the selected districts were grouped, if necessary, so that each secondary school or school group contained children of all ages between eleven and fifteen and children of both sexes. Once this had been done, all the primary schools in the selected districts were grouped up with secondary schools so that, within each district, there resulted a number of school groups each containing children of both sexes and of all ages from five to fifteen. The grouping of the primary schools was carried out using two criteria. First, to minimise travelling for the dentists at the examination stage, the schools were clustered geographically. Secondly, the schools were grouped so that large secondary schools had a proportionately higher number of primary schools linked to them than the smaller secondary schools. Once this grouping had taken place, one secondary school was

selected from each district with probability proportional to its size. Once a secondary school had been selected its attached primary schools were automatically selected.

It had been intended that each selected group of schools would provide one week's workload for a dentist but when the school groups were selected it was obvious that in some areas there would be too many schools for a dentist to visit in a week. We therefore reduced the number of schools the dentist would need to visit by randomly rejecting primary schools, so that the number of schools remaining in each group could all be visited in one week. We corrected for this random rejection of schools at the next stage when sampling individual children so that the sample remained self-weighting. To achieve this a constant number of secondary school children were selected from each school group. Using this number, a sampling interval was calculated for each secondary school. This same interval was used to sample the children in the connected primary schools (except in cases where some primary schools had been randomly rejected, in which case the sampling interval was reduced so as to select more primary school children in the schools that remained in the sample). OPCS interviewers visited the selected schools in November 1982 and sampled children from the school registers using calculated intervals.

The selection of the sample in Scotland differed only in the fact that the secondary schools were not initially allocated to local authority districts. Instead all secondary schools in Scotland were grouped in such a way that each resultant group contained children of all ages over ten and of both sexes. Thirty secondary schools (or school groups) were selected with probability proportional to size. Once these schools had been selected, the districts within which each was located were identified and within each of these districts primary schools were grouped up to secondary schools in the same way as in England and Wales. Again, all primary schools in the district were grouped to secondary schools to ensure that each had a chance of selection through being linked to a secondary school even though, in this case, we already knew the selected secondary school. (We did not, however, inform the staff who carried out the groupings which secondary school had been selected because it was felt this might affect the way they carried out the groupings.)

The sample in Northern Ireland was selected by the Department of Health and Social Services in Northern Ireland using a similar scheme to that used in Scotland. Twenty units were selected for the survey in Northern Ireland.

1.3 The administration
The sample of children for the survey were sampled from the school registers and dentally examined at school. Before the survey could take place there was a considerable amount of administrative work to be

carried out to request co-operation from those concerned in each of the stages.

Once the sample of districts had been selected in July 1982 we wrote to the Local Education Authorities that contained these districts to inform them about the survey and ask their permission to contact the selected schools. Once the schools had been selected we wrote again to the education authorities informing them of the schools in their area that would be involved. We then wrote to the schools themselves enclosing an information sheet about the survey and asking for their co-operation in the two stages of the survey. First, we wanted our interviewers to visit the schools in November to draw the sample from the school registers. Secondly, we had to arrange for the dentists to visit the schools to carry out the examinations. We wanted to give the schools as much notice as possible about the dentists' visits so, before we wrote to them we had devised a timetable for the dentists' visits to the schools (which were to be in January and February 1983), so that we could inform the schools of the day to expect the dental team. In the event, some schools contacted us to inform us that the day we had chosen would be inconvenient and so we were able to rearrange the timetables before the fieldwork period.

Each of the selected schools was visited in November 1982 by an interviewer working for Social Survey Division. At the school, the interviewer sampled through the school registers recording the name and date of birth of each of the selected children. For children whose parents were to be contacted by post to collect background information (see Section 1.6 below), the interviewer also recorded the home address of the child.

The parents of each of the selected children were informed about the survey and given the opportunity to say if they did not want their child to be included in the survey. Once the sample was selected, the interviewer left at the school a letter to be taken home by the selected children to inform their parents about the survey and asking them to contact the school if they did not wish their child to be included. Using a pre-carbonated pad, the interviewer made four copies of the sample list, one of which was sent to Social Survey Division and three left with the school. If any parents told the school that they did not wish their child to be included, the school marked their sheets accordingly and sent one copy to Social Survey Division so that the refusals could be deleted. One copy of the sample was given to the dental team when they arrived to carry out the examinations and one copy was retained by the school for their information.

We had designed the survey so that we put as small a burden of work on the schools as possible but, we did need them to carry out certain administrative tasks and we were very grateful for the high level of co-operation we received.

1.4 The dental examination team

In the 1973 Children's Dental Health Survey the dentists who worked on the survey were seconded from the Community Dental Service, and worked in the schools with a Social Survey interviewer who acted as the dental recorder during the examinations. In 1983 the dental examiners were again seconded from the Community Dental Service but it was also decided to ask for the secondment of a dental nurse to act as dental recorder in the schools.

On previous surveys the dental training had lasted for a week and involved two days of 'classroom' training, two days of practice examinations in local schools and a half-day calibration exercise. By the time of the 1983 survey, there was a body of dentists in the country who had worked on at least one of the previous national studies. It was therefore decided to utilise this past experience by using, as far as possible, dentists who had worked on one of the previous national surveys. In this way the training time could be reduced to the two days practice in schools and half-day calibration exercise with evening sessions to resolve any queries. The dental nurses joined the dentists for the second day of practice and for the calibration exercise.

Prior to the training courses the dentists and dental nurses were sent the examination criteria and a tape of example examinations so that they could familiarise themselves with the examination procedures and practise recording on the survey examination charts.

A total of 76 dentists were trained in Newcastle in two sessions during January 1983. The dentists were divided into regional teams each headed by a regional organiser who had taken part in the pilot study the previous autumn. The regional organisers were responsible for their team of dentists both at the training course and during the fieldwork period.

The dental teams started work on the Monday following their training course. Each group of schools was scheduled to be one week's work for a dentist. Some dentists had just one group of schools to visit while others had two or three weeks work. The dentists were also encouraged, if possible, to return to schools where there had been several absentees on the first visit in order to maximise the number of achieved examinations.

The majority of examinations were completed by mid-February 1983. Part of the sample had, however, been selected on one of the Scottish Islands and it was decided to delay the examinations there until April in case bad weather in February prevented the dental team either visiting or leaving the island.

1.5 The dental examination

The criteria for the dental examination were developed by the dental schools at Birmingham and Newcastle Universities. They were designed to collect information that could be compared directly with the information collected in the 1973 Survey. However in 1983, there

were certain topics in dental health that had not been relevant in 1973 but for which it was decided that information should be collected in 1983; for example the presence of fissure sealants and the presence of acid-etch restorations for traumatically damaged incisors.

In other areas of dental health, different methods of assessment had been developed since 1973 and it was decided to include some of these in the 1983 Survey. In particular, a section was included to measure the health of the gums using the criteria formulated by the World Health Organisation. The criteria used in the dental examination appear in the Appendix together with a copy of the examination chart.

1.6 The questionnaire

In the 1973 survey, interviewers from Social Survey Division interviewed the mothers of children aged five, eight, twelve and fourteen. (The reason the parents of fourteen year olds were interviewed rather than the parents of the fifteen year olds was because, in 1973, some fifteen year olds had left school and thus this age group was incomplete. In 1983, due to the change in the minimum school leaving age, the fifteen year old age group was complete.)

At the time of planning the 1983 survey it was decided, for reasons of economy, to explore the possibility of collecting background information about the children in the sample by post. A postal questionnaire cannot collect the same amount of detailed information that can be collected via a personal interview. However, previous social survey work on a survey of mothers' experiences of breast feeding which had been carried out in 1975 by a personal interview[2] and in 1980 by means of a postal questionnaire[3] gave us an indication of the types of questions that could be answered adequately by means of a postal inquiry.

The use of a postal questionnaire was piloted in the autumn of 1983 and resulted in the decision being made to use this form of data collection at the main stage.

When the interviewers visited the schools to carry out the sampling of children for the survey (see Section 1.3) they recorded the home address of all the children who would be aged five, eight, twelve and fifteen by 31st December 1982. Questionnaires were sent by post to the parents of these children at the end of January (provided the parents had not said that they did not wish their child to be examined). Those parents who had not replied by mid-February were sent a reminder letter. A further reminder was sent to those who had not replied by end of February and in mid-March Social Survey interviewers visited those parents from whom we had still not received a completed questionnaire to collect incompleted questionnaires from them.

As in 1973 we were only interested in collecting background information from children who had been dentally examined. Parents who had said that they did not wish their child to be examined were excluded from

the initial mailing. It was not known, at that time, however, which other children had not been examined for other reasons, such as absence from school, and so parents of these children were sent questionnaires at the initial stage. They were not, however, included in the reminder system.

A copy of the questionnaire is given in the Appendix E.

1.7 The response
The dental health survey relied on co-operation at several stages before the children could be examined. First, the local authorities were asked permission to involve schools in their areas and we were gratified that this permission was given in all cases. Second, the individual schools had to give their consent to us involving their children. In a few cases, a school was unwilling to co-operate and it was calculated that 3% of the potential sample would have been selected from these schools (Table 1.1). Once the children had been sampled, their parents were sent letters about the survey and asked to inform the schools if they did not wish their child to be examined. A further 2% of children were excluded for this reason.

The sampling of the children took place in the school term prior to that in which the dental examinations took place, and in this period some children had moved school and thus could not be examined. This accounted for a further 2% of the sample.

Another reason for not examining selected children was if they were absent each time the dentists called.

Table 1.1 The response

The dental examination		
Sample	22,375	100%
Children not examined due to non-co-operation of school	590	3%
Parent unwilling for child to be examined	541	2%
Child left the school	419	2%
Child absent all visits	1,065	5%
		12%
Successfully examined		88%
The postal questionnaire		
Sample (Parents with children of the relevant age who had been examined)	6,869	100%
Returned by post office	197	3%
Never returned	157	2%
		5%
Completed postal questionnaires returned		95%

The dental team had been given a very heavy workload which permitted very little time to recall at schools, because we had wished to keep the time period that they were seconded to us as short as possible. A loss through absenteeism had therefore been expected. In all, 5% of the sample were not examined through being away from school at each visit.

Taking all these stages into account, it can be seen that the response rate to the examination stage of the survey was 88%.

Most of the children who were not examined were withdrawn from the sample before the time of the examination, due to reasons such as school or parental non co-operation. Of the children that were in the sample at the time when the survey dental examiner visited the school (20,825) successful examinations were carried out in 95% of cases.

The response rate to the postal questionnaire was high, boosted by the fact that several reminder letters were used and interviewers collected questionnaires from households where there had been no response by post. In the examination stage of the survey, 6,869 children aged five, eight, twelve and fifteen were examined and we received completed questionnaires from the parents of 6,515, a response rate of 95%.

1.8 The presentation of the results
The two main aims of the 1983 survey were to provide data for comparison with that collected in England and Wales on the 1973 Children's Dental Health Survey and to provide information about the state of children's dental health in the constituent countries of the United Kingdom in 1983. In addition to the data collected from children of all ages at the dental examination, background information was collected from the parents of children of four ages.

In order to present information separately for Wales, Scotland and Northern Ireland an enhanced sample was drawn in these countries, and when results are presented for the constituent countries it is on these enhanced sample sizes that the figures are based. When results are presented for England and Wales together or for the United Kingdom as a whole the results for the constituent countries are down weighted so that they contribute to the overall figures in their correct proportions.

References
[1] J E Todd, *Children's dental health in England and Wales 1973*. HMSO (1975).
[2] Jean Martin. *Infant feeding 1975*. HMSO (1978).
[3] Jean Martin and Janet Monk, *Infant feeding 1980*. OPCS (1982).

2 Missing deciduous teeth, deciduous decay experience and the eruption of the permanent teeth.

2.1 Introduction

The survey of children's dental health was carried out in January and February 1983 and in November of that year an OPCS monitor giving the preliminary results from the survey was published. It showed that the proportion of five year olds in England and Wales with some filled teeth or some actively decayed teeth had decreased from 71% in 1973 to 48% in 1983 and that the average number of filled or decayed deciduous teeth in five year olds had decreased from 3.4 teeth in 1973 to 1.7 teeth in 1983. Among fifteen year olds in England and Wales the proportions with some permanent teeth that were decayed, filled or missing due to decay were similar in 1973 and 1983 but the average number of permanent teeth that were decayed, filled or missing due to decay decreased from 8.4 teeth in 1973 to 5.6 teeth in 1983.

The preliminary results also showed that in 1983 there was considerable variation in the state of dental health between children in the constituent countries of the United Kingdom. Among five year olds for example the average number of deciduous teeth that were filled or decayed varied from 1.6 among children in England to 2.6 among children in Wales, 3.2 among children in Scotland and 3.7 among children in Northern Ireland.

Among fifteen year olds the average number of permanent teeth that were decayed, filled or missing due to decay varied between 5.6 teeth among children in England, 6.7 among children in Wales, 8.4 among children in Scotland and 9.2 among children in Northern Ireland.

In this report we expand on these initial results as well as presenting information on the other topics covered in the survey. However before presenting the main survey findings we begin in this chapter by making an assessment of the contribution made by missing deciduous teeth to the total decay experience of the deciduous dentition. It is often difficult to tell, once a deciduous tooth is absent, the reason for its loss, and it is impossible to tell whether or not it had decay experience prior to its loss. This is particularly true among older children with a mixed dentition because one cannot predict at exactly what age the deciduous dentition will naturally exfoliate. In the survey dental examination the same methodology was to be used for all children regardless of age. Consequently, as in the 1973 survey, the dental examiners were not asked to assess the reason for the absence of deciduous teeth. It is possible however to make various assumptions based on the child's age and dental condition and in this chapter we make some estimates of the numbers of deciduous teeth lost due to decay, or diseased before exfoliation, and thus estimate the total decay experience of the deciduous dentition.

Also in this chapter we look at the retention of deciduous teeth and the eruption patterns of the permanent dentition, comparing the situation in 1973 with that in 1983.

2.2 Total decay experience for the deciduous dentition among five year olds

Five year olds were the youngest age group covered in the survey and, for that age group, there are various assumptions that can be made concerning the reason for loss of the deciduous teeth and their health prior to loss, according to which type of tooth is lost and the dental health of the surrounding teeth. These assumptions (which are the same as those made in the 1973 survey report) give the following estimates of total deciduous decay experience:

Estimate I   Assume all missing deciduous teeth were extracted due to decay or were diseased before they exfoliated.

Estimate II   Assume all missing deciduous teeth (except the lower central incisors) were extracted due to decay or were diseased before they exfoliated.

Assume missing lower central incisors had exfoliated without being diseased unless any of the lower anterior teeth were present and diseased or either canine was missing; in which case assume the missing lower central incisors had been decayed.

Estimate III   Assume all missing deciduous teeth (except incisors) were extracted due to decay or were diseased before they exfoliated.

Assume missing upper incisors had exfoliated without being diseased unless 3 or 4 of the upper incisors were absent without any eruption of the permanent dentition.

Assume missing lower incisors had exfoliated without being diseased unless any of the lower anterior teeth were present and diseased or either canine was missing; in which case assume the missing lower incisors had been decayed.

Estimate IV   Assume all missing deciduous teeth (except incisors) were extracted due to decay or were diseased before exfoliation. Assume missing incisors were naturally exfoliated with no decay experience.

Estimate V   Assume all missing deciduous teeth were naturally exfoliated with no decay experience.

Using these assumptions we can calculate the proportion of five year olds in England and Wales who have or have had some decay experience of their deciduous dentition (that is, some actively decayed teeth, some filled teeth, some teeth missing due to decay or some teeth which had naturally exfoliated but were previously diseased) and compare these proportions with the estimates made in 1973 (Table 2.1).

Table 2.1   Estimates of the proportion of five year olds with deciduous decay experience in England and Wales in 1973 and in 1983

Estimate	Proportion of five year olds with decay experience	
	1973	1983
Estimate I	79%	60%
Estimate II	74%	53%
Estimate III	72%	49%
Estimate IV	72%	49%
Estimate V	71%	48%
Base	*952*	*719*

Under each of the estimates the proportion of children with some decay experience was lower in 1983 than in 1973. Under Estimate I (all missing teeth previously decayed) the proportion of children with decay experience was relatively high (60%) in 1983. However, Estimate I was made to show the opposite end of the range of assumptions to Estimate V. It is clearly not a realistic assumption as it is known that some children do lose their deciduous incisors naturally before the age of six. Similarly, Estimate V is unlikely to be a realistic estimate as it assumes that not one lost deciduous tooth

had decay experience. However, the more realistic assumptions give a proportion of children with some decay experience very much nearer to the figure Estimate V gives than the figure Estimate I gives. In 1973 it was concluded that Estimate III was likely to be the most accurate; that is that all lost posterior teeth are presumed to have decay experience and missing incisors are presumed to have been decayed only if there was current decay experience in that part of the mouth. Under this assumption it can be seen that 49% of five year olds in England and Wales in 1983 had some decay experience of their deciduous dentition.

Table 2.2 shows the average number of deciduous teeth with decay experience among five year olds in England and Wales in 1973 and 1983. Estimate V (which assumes no loss through decay of the primary dentition and no prior decay on naturally exfoliated teeth) shows the average number of filled and decayed deciduous teeth. Taking the most realistic assumption (Estimate III) it can be seen that in 1973 this increased the average decay experience from the most optimistic estimate (V) by 0.7 teeth in 1973. In 1983, however, the difference between the average number of teeth with decay experience under Estimate V and Estimate III was just 0.2 teeth.

Table 2.3 shows the proportion of five year olds in the constituent countries of the United Kingdom with some decay experience of the deciduous teeth. It can be seen that moving from Estimate V which assumes no decay experience of missing deciduous teeth to Estimate III which assumes missing posterior deciduous teeth to have been diseased and missing anterior deciduous teeth to have been diseased if there is evidence of disease in that part of the mouth, increases the proportion of children with some decay experience by just one percentage point in each of the countries except Northern Ireland, where it increases from 74% under Estimate V to 78% under Estimate III.

Table 2.4 shows the average number of deciduous teeth with decay experience, for five year olds in the constituent countries of the United Kingdom. The least variation between the estimates made of total deciduous decay experience is seen among five year olds in England. Even under the most pessimistic assumption, that all missing teeth were previously diseased, the average number of deciduous teeth with decay experience is lower in England than the most optimistic estimate of the average number of deciduous teeth with known decay experience in any of the other countries.

Table 2.2   Estimated average number of deciduous teeth with decay experience among five year olds in England and Wales in 1973 and 1983

Estimate	Average number of teeth with decay experience	
	1973	1983
Estimate I	4.6	2.4
Estimate II	4.2	2.0
Estimate III	4.0	1.8
Estimate IV	3.9	1.8
Estimate V	3.3	1.6
Base	*952*	*719*

Table 2.3   Estimated proportion of five year olds with decay experience in their deciduous dentition in United Kingdom in 1983

Estimate	England	Wales	Scotland	Northern Ireland	United Kingdom
Estimate I	59%	75%	80%	83%	62%
Estimate II	52%	70%	78%	80%	55%
Estimate III	48%	67%	75%	78%	52%
Estimate IV	48%	67%	75%	78%	52%
Estimate V	47%	66%	74%	74%	51%
Base	*671*	*190*	*319*	*198*	*804*

Table 2.4 Estimated average number of deciduous teeth with decay experience among five year olds in United Kingdom

Estimate	England	Wales	Scotland	Northern Ireland	United Kingdom
Estimate I	2.3	3.8	4.6	5.3	2.7
Estimate II	1.9	3.4	4.1	4.9	2.2
Estimate III	1.8	3.1	3.9	4.5	2.1
Estimate IV	1.8	3.0	3.9	4.5	2.0
Estimate V	1.6	2.6	3.2	3.7	1.8
Base	*671*	*190*	*319*	*198*	*804*

It can be seen that, when the average number of deciduous teeth with decay experience estimated first by III (assuming all missing back teeth were previously decayed and that missing incisors were previously decayed only if there was current decay experience in that part of the mouth) and then by IV (assuming that all missing back teeth had been previously decayed and that all missing incisors had exfoliated without decay), there was very little difference. This was true in each of the countries.

If we assume that Estimate III is the most reasonable estimate for the five year olds, it can be seen that in the United Kingdom as a whole there was an average of 2.1 deciduous teeth that had, at some time, been decayed while there was an average of 1.8 deciduous teeth that were decayed or filled at the time of the examination. Thus, in the United Kingdom, the contribution made to the total decay experience of deciduous teeth by the teeth which were missing at the time of the examination was small. This difference was also small among five year olds in England, but in the other countries the estimated contribution to the total decay experience of the deciduous teeth from teeth that were missing was higher. Again, if we assume Estimate III to be the most accurate estimation for five year olds, it can be seen that the missing deciduous teeth contribute to total decay experience 0.5 teeth among five year olds in Wales, 0.7 teeth among five year olds in Scotland and 0.8 teeth among five year olds in Northern Ireland.

2.3 Estimated deciduous decay experience for children aged six to eight

As children grow older more of their deciduous teeth exfoliate naturally and it is thus more difficult to make assumptions about the health of the missing deciduous teeth. We did, however, think that it was useful to make an estimate of total deciduous decay experience for children aged up to eight years.

We saw in the previous section that it made very little difference to the estimate of known decay experience of the five year olds whether we assumed that all missing deciduous teeth apart from incisors were lost due to decay (or were decayed before exfoliation) and that the missing incisors had been decayed if there was some evidence of decay in the same part of the mouth (Estimate III) or whether we assumed only that the posterior missing teeth had been decayed and that missing incisors were decay free when they exfoliated (Estimate IV). Among the older children it is likely that a higher proportion of deciduous incisors will have exfoliated naturally without disease, and so we assume only that the missing deciduous molars and canines were previously diseased. Among the older of these children it is likely that there will have been some loss of deciduous canines and molars which have exfoliated without decay so our estimates of total deciduous decay experience show a maximum estimate.

Table 2.5 shows the estimated average number of deciduous teeth that have or have had decay experience among children aged six to eight and the average number of decayed and filled deciduous teeth at the time of the dental examination. Thus the contribution to the total decay experience of the deciduous dentition made by teeth that are no longer present in the mouth can be seen.

There are some very large national variations both in the total decay experience and in the contribution made by the missing deciduous teeth. For example among seven year olds there was an estimated average number of deciduous teeth with known decay experience of 3.2 in England, 3.4 in Wales, 5.0 in Scotland and 5.3 in Northern Ireland. Thus it can be seen that among seven year olds in England it was estimated that 0.9 deciduous teeth were missing due to decay or had been diseased before exfoliation compared with 1.0 teeth in Wales, 2.0 teeth in Scotland and 1.8 teeth in Northern Ireland.

Table 2.5 Average number of deciduous teeth with decay experience and average number of deciduous teeth decayed or filled at the time of the survey dental examination

Age	England		Wales		Scotland		Northern Ireland		United Kingdom	
	Decayed or filled	Estimated total experience	Decayed or filled	Estimated total experience	Decayed or filled	Estimated total experience	Decayed or filled	Estimated total experience	Decayed or filled	Estimated total experience
6	1.9	2.4	2.7	3.3	3.2	4.3	3.0	4.2	2.1	2.7
7	2.3	3.2	2.4	3.4	3.0	5.0	3.5	5.3	2.4	3.4
8	2.2	3.9	2.8	4.9	3.3	6.4	3.0	6.1	2.3	4.2

For bases see Appendix A

2.4 The eruption of the permanent dentition

In this section we look at the changes that took place in the ages at which different permanent teeth erupted into the mouth, in England and Wales, between 1973 and 1983.

Figures 2.1 and 2.2 show, for individual permanent tooth types in the upper and lower jaws, the proportion of children in each age group for whom that tooth had erupted, for children in England and Wales in both 1973 and 1983. (Because the figures were so similar for the right side and the left side of the jaw, we present those relating to the left side only.)

Looking first at the upper jaw (Figure 2.1) it can be seen that the eruption patterns for the permanent incisors and canines were the same in 1973 and 1983. In the case of the first premolar, however, there was a slight variation between 1973 and 1983 in the proportion of children in each age group for whom this tooth had erupted. Although in each of the individual age groups none of the differences were statistically significant, there was an indication that the upper first premolar was erupting at a slightly later age in 1983 than in 1973, for in each of the age groups up to the age of twelve a slightly lower proportion of children in 1983 than in 1973 had this tooth erupted.

This was also true for the upper second premolar, and in this case the differences were larger. For example, among eleven year olds in England and Wales in 1973, 61% had their permanent upper left second premolar compared with 50% of eleven year olds in 1983.

There was no difference between the eruption patterns of the upper first molar in 1973 and 1983 but in the case of the upper second molar there was in each age group, a slightly lower proportion of children in 1983 for whom the second molar had erupted, but these differences were not statistically significant.

In the lower jaw (Figure 2.2) there were no differences between 1973 and 1983 in the eruption patterns of the permanent incisors but there was a very slight indication of a later age for the eruption of the lower canine in 1983 than in 1973.

There was no difference in the eruption patterns of the lower first premolar between 1973 and 1983. In the case of the lower second premolar, in each of the age groups, a slightly lower proportion of children in 1983 than in 1973 had this tooth erupted, but these differences were not as large as in the case of the upper second premolar.

There was no real difference between the eruption patterns of the lower permanent molars in 1973 and 1983.

There were some indications of a later eruption of the upper first premolar, the upper second molar, the lower canine and the lower second premolar, but the only significant differences in the eruption patterns of

permanent teeth occurred in the case of the upper second premolar.

A possible reason for a later eruption of the permanent dentition is that deciduous teeth were being retained in the jaw for a longer period due to the decrease in dental decay and thereby affecting the timing of the eruption of their permanent successors. To see to what extent later retention of the deciduous dentition was associated with the erruption of the permanent dentition we look in Figures 2.3 and 2.4 at the proportions of children who retained certain teeth at different ages in 1973 and 1983.

In the upper jaw (Figure 2.3) it can be seen that there was very little difference in the proportions of children of different ages in 1973 and 1983 who still had their deciduous incisors or canines. However, in the case of the first and second deciduous molars (which precede the first and second premolars) there was a significant change over the ten year period in the proportions of children retaining these teeth. For example, in 1973, 74% of eight year olds retained their upper left first deciduous molar compared with 86% of eight year olds in 1983. Among ten year olds, 54% still had their upper left second deciduous molar in 1973 compared with 66% in 1983.

In the lower jaw (Figure 2.4), there was again no difference in the proportion of children of different ages in 1973 and 1983 who still had their deciduous molars and canines. There were, however, some large differences in the proportions of children of different ages who retained their lower deciduous molars, particularly in the case of the lower second molar. For example, in 1973 67% of eight year olds retained their lower left second molar compared with 87% of eight year olds in 1983.

Thus it would seem that the overall retention of the deciduous teeth to a later age in 1983 due to the fall in the caries rate, may be associated with the later eruption of the permanent teeth. However, it cannot be said that the former completely emplains the latter. It was shown, for example, that of the second premolars, the largest change in eruption patterns that had occurred was with regard to the upper second premolar. However, in the case of deciduous second molars, the largest changes in retention was found in the lower jaw. It was also shown that the upper second permanent molar seemed, on average, to be erupting at a later age in 1983 than in 1973, and yet there is no deciduous tooth preceding the second permanent molar. The second molars erupt comparatively late in a child's life and by the time they erupt some children may have already lost their first permanent molars because of decay. It may be that if the first molar is lost, the second molar erupts earlier than it would have done if the first molar had still been present. Figure 2.5 shows the proportions of children in 1973 and in 1983 who had lost their upper or lower left first permanent molar. It can be seen that a higher proportion of children in 1973 than in 1983 had had their upper left

permanent molar extracted due to decay and this might have been a reason for the slightly earlier eruption of the upper second permanent molar in 1973 than in 1983. However, Figure 2.5 also shows that there were higher proportions of children in 1973 than in 1983 who had lost a lower first permanent molar due to decay yet it was shown that there was little difference between 1973 and 1983 in the eruption patterns of the lower second permanent molar.

Generally, any changes in the eruption patterns of the permanent teeth between 1973 and 1983 were small, but there did appear to be a tendency towards the later eruption of certain of the permanent tooth types and that these changes in eruption patterns may be associated with the changes seen in the age to which children retain their posterior deciduous teeth.

2.5 Summary

The proportion of five year olds in England and Wales who had decayed or filled deciduous teeth at the time of the survey dental examination fell from 71% in 1973 to 48% in 1983. The average number of deciduous teeth showing evidence of decay experience was 3.4 in 1973 and this had fallen to 1.7 in 1983. When allowance is made for the possible disease experience of deciduous teeth that were already missing among five year olds then the proportion of five year olds with decay experience fell from 72% in 1973 to 49% in 1983. The average number of teeth estimated to have had some decay experience, allowing for the condition of the missing deciduous teeth was 4.0 in 1973 dropping to 1.8 in 1983. The effect of the adjustment for the possible disease experience of the missing deciduous teeth is greater on the average number of teeth affected than on the proportion of children with some decay experience because most children whose missing deciduous teeth were deemed to have been decayed before they were lost also had some evidence of decay or treatment for decay in their remaining deciduous teeth.

A higher proportion of children retained their deciduous teeth, especially their deciduous molars for longer in 1983 than had been the case in 1973 and there was some evidence that some posterior teeth in the permanent dentition were erupting later in 1983 than had been the case ten years earlier.

Figure 2.1 Permanent tooth eruption patterns by age in 1973 and 1983 - upper jaw

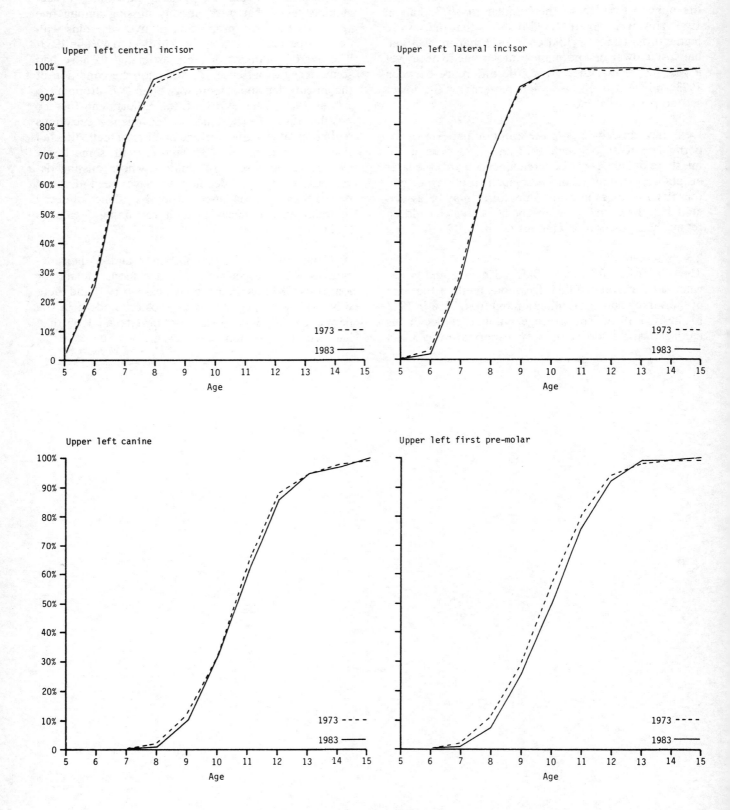

Figure 2.1 contd

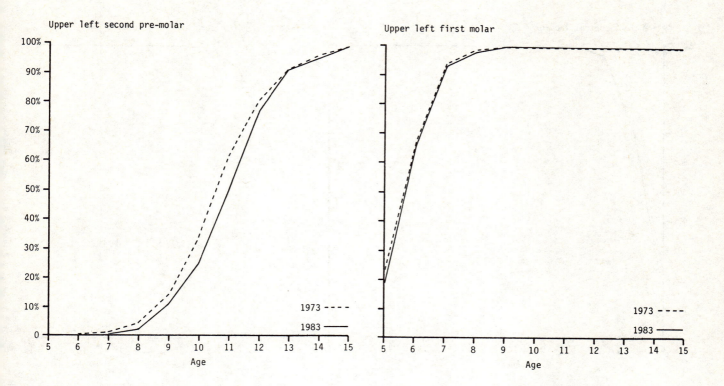

Upper left second pre-molar

Upper left first molar

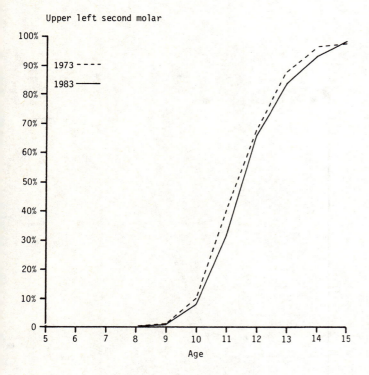

Upper left second molar

11

Figure 2.2 Permanent tooth eruption patterns by age in 1973 and 1983 - lower jaw

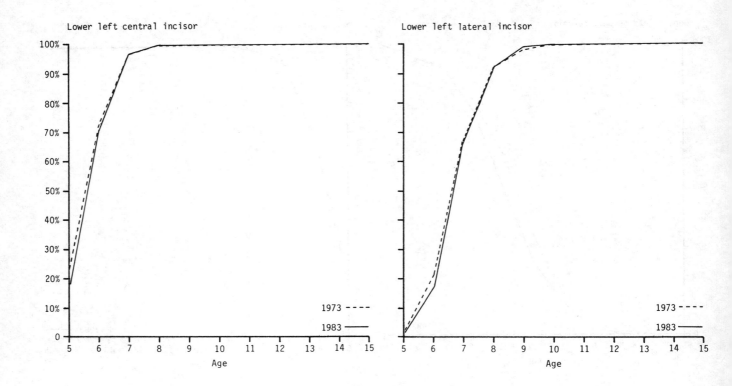

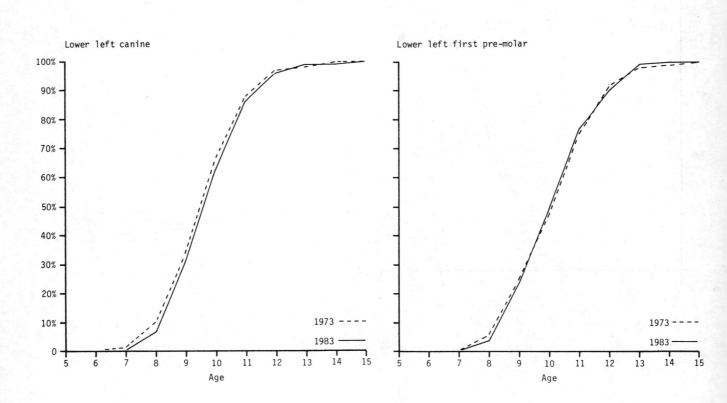

Figure 2.2 contd

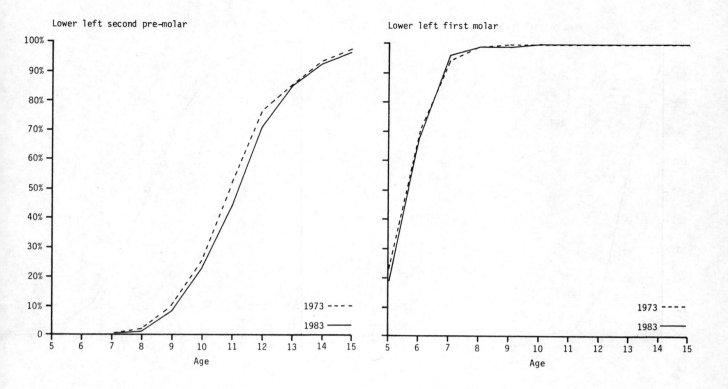

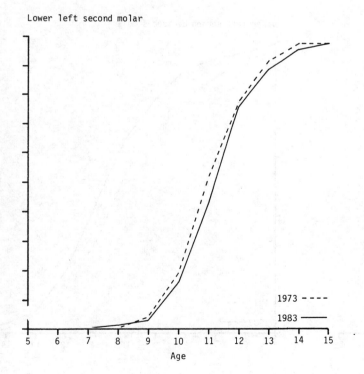

Figure 2.3 Proportion of deciduous teeth present by age in 1973 and 1983 - upper jaw

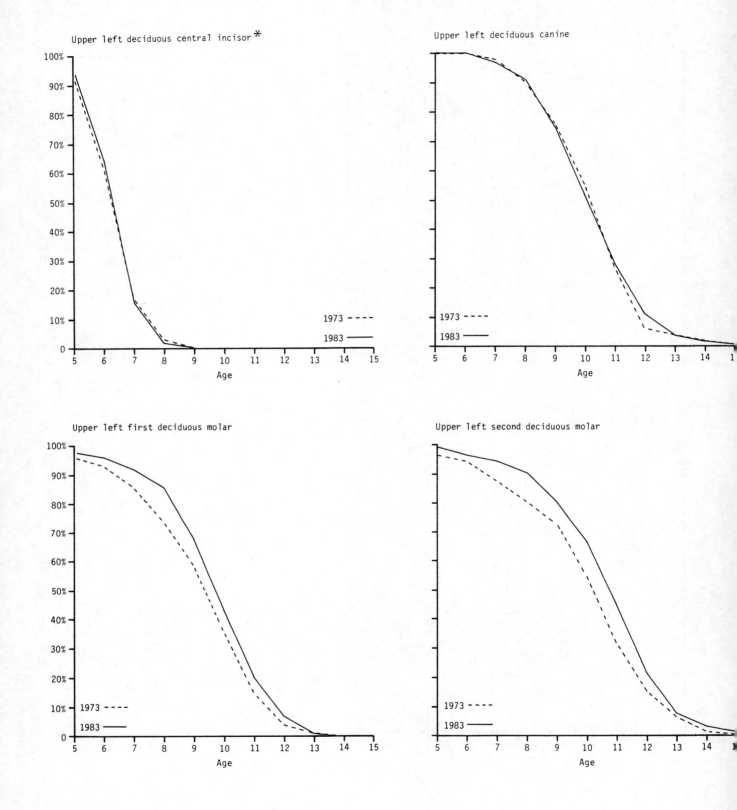

*The proportions of upper left deciduous lateral incisors present in 1983 were similar to the proportions present in 1973 and thus the figure is not presented for this tooth

Figure 2.4 Proportion of deciduous teeth present by age in 1973 and 1983 - lower jaw

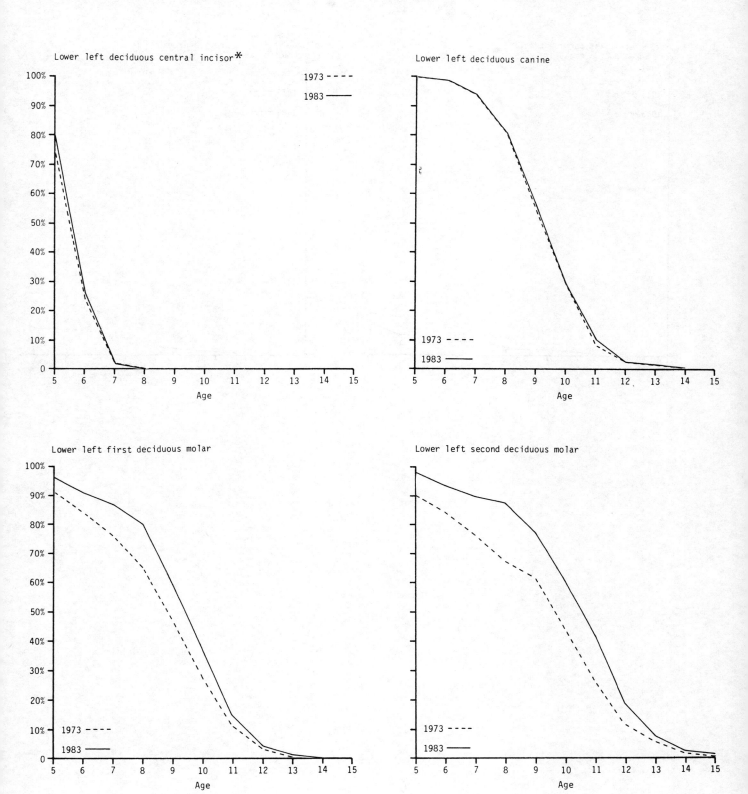

*The proportions of lower left deciduous lateral incisors present in 1983 were similar to the proportions present in 1973 and thus the figure is not presented for this tooth

Figure 2.5 The proportion of children whose first permanent molar had been extracted due to decay

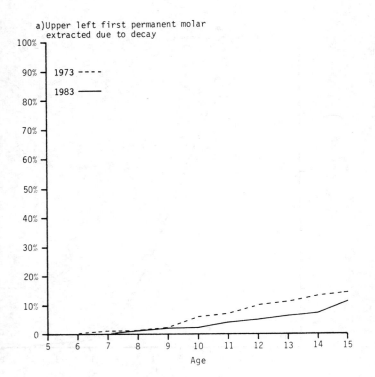

a)Upper left first permanent molar
   extracted due to decay

1973 ----
1983 ——

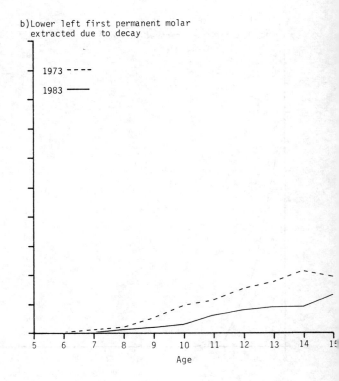

b)Lower left first permanent molar
   extracted due to decay

1973 ----
1983 ——

3 The condition of children's teeth in the United Kingdom in 1983

3.1 Introduction

The major part of the survey dental examination was the assessment of the decay experience of the children's teeth and this measurement is presented in this chapter for both the deciduous and permanent dentition in order to see the variation between the constituent countries of the United Kingdom. Decay experience is defined as teeth which are currently decayed (including teeth which have been previously filled but are now in need of further treatment), teeth which are filled but otherwise sound and teeth which have been extracted because they have been decayed.

Any assessment of the total decay experience of children is complicated by the natural exfoliation patterns of the deciduous teeth in that once a deciduous tooth is lost from the mouth it is impossible to know whether or not that tooth was previously decayed. As the deciduous teeth exfoliate at different times in different children it is also very difficult to know when a deciduous tooth is missing, whether it has naturally exfoliated or whether it had been lost due to decay. We did not ask the dentists to record an assessment as to the reason for the loss of a deciduous tooth and so in this and later chapters, for the primary dentition, we use solely the measures of current decay and restorative treatment. In the previous chapter, however, we looked at some of the estimates that could be made of the total deciduous decay experience. It was seen that under the most realistic assumption concerning missing deciduous teeth, the proportion of five year olds in the United Kingdom with some deciduous decay experience was one percentage point higher than the proportion of five year olds with some decayed or filled deciduous teeth. The average number of teeth with deciduous decay experience among five year olds in the United Kingdom was estimated at 0.3 teeth higher than the average number of decayed or filled deciduous teeth. This figure varied between five year olds in the constituent countries of the United Kingdom from 0.2 teeth among children in England, 0.3 teeth among children in Wales, 0.7 teeth among children in Scotland and 0.8 teeth among children in Northern Ireland. These figures can be borne in mind when assessing the variations in disease experience presented in this chapter.

3.2 Active decay

Active decay is a measure of current treatment need. Figure 3.1* shows how the proportion of children with some active decay in their deciduous teeth varies between the constituent countries of the United Kingdom. Overall, in the United Kingdom, this proportion increases gradually with age until the age of nine.

Among the older children it decreases sharply as deciduous teeth are lost. It can be seen, however, that there are very large differences in this proportion between the constituent countries of the United Kingdom. Among five year olds, for example, 37% of children from England had some active decay of their deciduous teeth at the time of the survey dental examination compared with 48% of five year olds from Wales, 66% from Scotland and 68% from Northern Ireland.

Generally Scotland and Northern Ireland were in a less favourable position and England was in the most favourable position. In the age range five to eight Wales had a lower proportion of children with some active decay in the deciduous dentition than Scotland or Northern Ireland but in the older age groups there was little difference between children from Wales and children from Scotland in the proportion with some active decay.

There were very large differences in the proportion of children with some active decay in their permanent dentition between the countries of the United Kingdom (Figure 3.2). There was a higher proportion of children with active decay in their permanent dentition in Northern Ireland than in any of the other countries. In fact, in the ages up to thirteen there were proportionately approximately twice as many children from Northern Ireland with active decay as from England. Generally, the children from England showed the lowest proportion with some active decay in their permanent teeth although there was little difference between the children from England and the children from Wales in the younger ages. The children from Scotland, generally, had a lower proportion with some decay experience in the permanent dentition than children from Northern Ireland but higher than children from England or Wales. For example among thirteen year olds, there were 64% of children from Northern Ireland with active decay of the permanent dentition, 51% from Scotland, 40% from Wales and 31% from England.

Figures 3.3 and 3.4 show the average number of deciduous and permanent teeth with some active decay. The comparative differences between the averages in the countries are similar to those seen between the proportions of children with some active decay.

---

* The tables on which all the figures in this report are based appear in the Appendix Table section at the back of the report and a summary table is (Table 3.11) included at the end of this chapter.

Figure 3.1 Proportion of children with some active decay in the deciduous dentition in UK in 1983

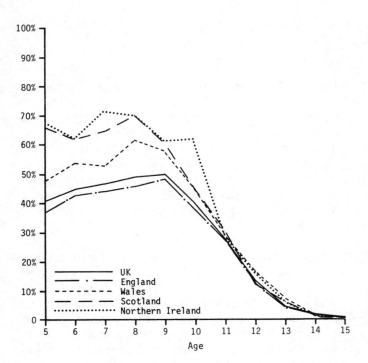

Figure 3.2 Proportion of children with some active decay in the permanent dentition in UK in 1983

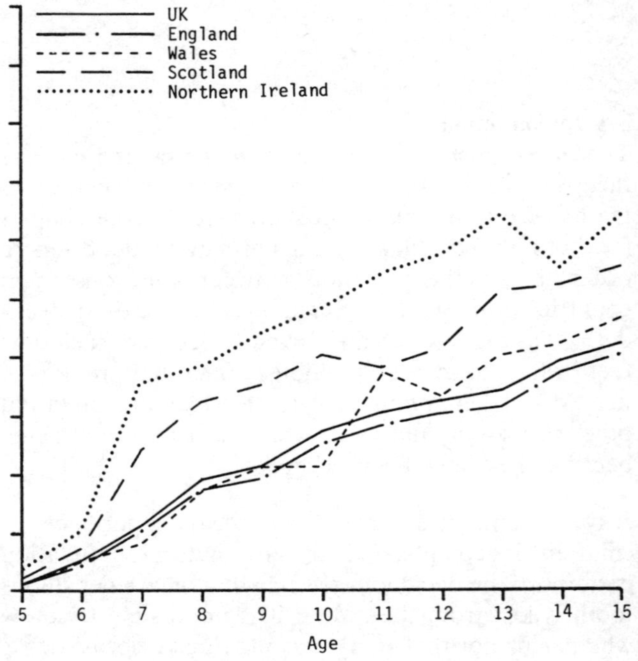

Figure 3.3 Average number of deciduous teeth with active decay in UK in 1983

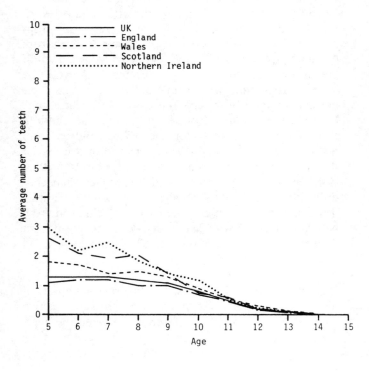

Figure 3.4 Average number of permanent teeth with active decay in UK in 1983

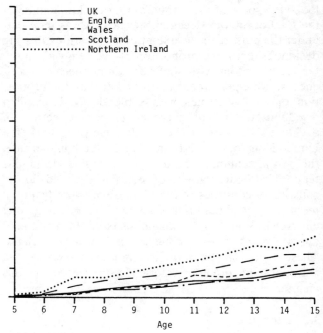

There was a particularly large variation in the average number of actively decayed deciduous teeth among five year olds. This figure was 1.1 teeth among five year olds in England, 1.8 teeth in Wales, 2.6 teeth in Scotland and 3.0 teeth among five year olds in Northern Ireland. Among the older children there was considerable variation between the countries in the average number of actively decayed permanent teeth. In each of the older age groups the average was at least twice as high in Northern Ireland as it was in England. Generally there was a lower average in Scotland than in Northern Ireland, and a still lower average in Wales, with children in England having the lowest average number of actively decayed permanent teeth. Among thirteen year olds, for example, the average number of actively decayed permanent teeth varied from 1.8 in Northern Ireland to 1.3 in Scotland, 0.9 in Wales and 0.6 in England.

3.3 Filled (otherwise sound) teeth

Teeth which have been filled represent a measure of past decay experience which has been treated with the aim of conserving the natural dentition. The decision to treat dental disease by restorative treatment may vary according to whether or not the disease affects the permanent or deciduous dentition. In the case of a permanent tooth, fillings are clearly preferable to extractions if the natural dentition is valued, because a lost permanent tooth will not be replaced. In the case of a decayed deciduous tooth the decision on whether or not to fill the tooth may be affected by the knowledge that the tooth will be lost naturally at some point.

Figure 3.5 shows the proportion of children with some filled (otherwise sound) deciduous teeth. This propor-

tion increased with age until the age of nine (from 23% of five year olds in the United Kingdom to 49% of nine year olds) and thereafter decreased. Among the youngest children, the lowest proportion with some filled teeth was among children in England (22%) and the highest among children in Wales (35%). In both Scotland and Northern Ireland, 26% of five year olds had some filled deciduous teeth.

Generally, Northern Ireland had a low proportion of children with some filled deciduous teeth and though there was little difference in the proportions between Northern Ireland and England in the younger age groups, in the age range nine to twelve, there was a substantially lower proportion of children with some filled deciduous teeth in Northern Ireland than in England. In fact, after the age of eight, England changes its position relative to the other countries. While among the younger children from England there was a relatively low proportion of children with filled deciduous teeth, among the older children there was a relatively high proportion. It would seem therefore that in England the decision to fill a deciduous tooth when it is diseased is taken more often than is the case in the other countries, particularly Scotland and Northern Ireland. We saw, in Chapter 2 that, in these latter two countries there was a much higher element of deciduous decay experience coming from missing deciduous teeth than was the case in England.

Figure 3.6 shows the proportions of children with some filled (otherwise sound) permanent teeth which are seen to increase very sharply with age. Generally the highest proportion of children with some filled permanent teeth was found in Scotland. In the age groups up

Figure 3.5 Proportion of children with some filled teeth in the deciduous dentition in UK in 1983

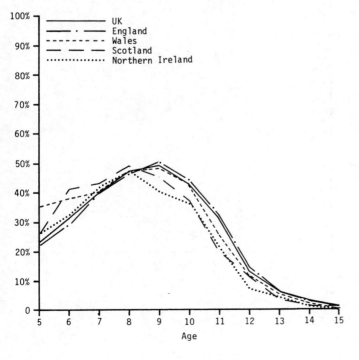

Figure 3.6 Proportion of children with some filled teeth in the permanent dentition in UK in 1983

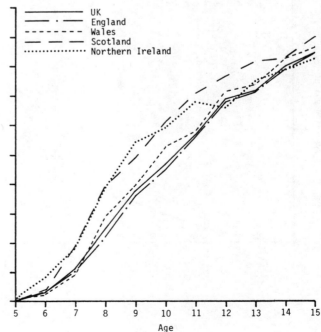

to eleven there was little difference between this proportion among children in Scotland and children in Northern Ireland. In the older age groups, however, there were lower proportions of children in Northern Ireland than in Scotland with some filled permanent teeth, and, in fact, in these older age groups there was little difference in this proportion between children in Northern Ireland, England and Wales. Although, generally, the lowest proportions of children with some filled permanent teeth were found in England, in the majority of age groups the differences between the proportions in England and the proportions in Wales were minimal.

Table 3.1 and Figure 3.7 show the variation in the average number of filled teeth between the countries of the United Kingdom. It can be seen that there was virtually no difference, between the countries, in the average number of filled deciduous teeth.

Table 3.1 Average number of deciduous teeth which were filled (otherwise sound) in the United Kingdom

Age	England	Wales	Scotland	Northern Ireland	United Kingdom
5	0.5	0.8	0.6	0.7	0.5
6	0.7	1.0	1.1	0.8	0.8
7	1.1	1.0	1.1	1.1	1.1
8	1.2	1.3	1.3	1.2	1.2
9	1.2	1.2	1.1	1.0	1.2
10	1.0	1.0	0.7	0.8	1.0
11	0.7	0.5	0.4	0.4	0.6
12	0.2	0.2	0.2	0.1	0.2
13	0.1	0.1	—	—	0.1
14	—	—	—	—	—
15	—	—	—	—	—

For bases see Appendix A

There was however variation in the average number of filled permanent teeth (Figure 3.7) with children from Scotland and Northern Ireland having a higher average number of filled permanent teeth than children from England and Wales. Among the older children the differences between these countries in the average number of filled permanent teeth were large, ranging from 5.8 teeth in Scotland and Northern Ireland to 4.8 teeth among children in Wales and 4.2 teeth among children in England. The higher average number of filled teeth in Scotland and Northern Ireland reflect the higher prevalence of dental decay that was noted in Section 3.2 above.

3.4 Missing teeth

The most serious effect of tooth decay is when a tooth has to be extracted because of decay and this is particularly serious in the case of permanent teeth. As explained above in Section 3.1, the assessment of the reason for loss of the deciduous teeth is complicated due to the natural exfoliation of the primary dentition. As we wished to use the same dental examination criteria for all the children in the survey we did not ask the dental examiner to record the reason for loss of the deciduous teeth but we have made certain estimates of the number of deciduous teeth which were not present which may have previously been decayed. These findings are presented in Chapter 2. In this section results are shown for permanent teeth that had been extracted due to decay, which were recorded by the dental examiner at the time of the examination.

Figure 3.7 Average number of permanent teeth which were filled (otherwise sound) in the UK in 1983

Figure 3.8 Proportion of children with some permanent teeth missing due to decay in 1983

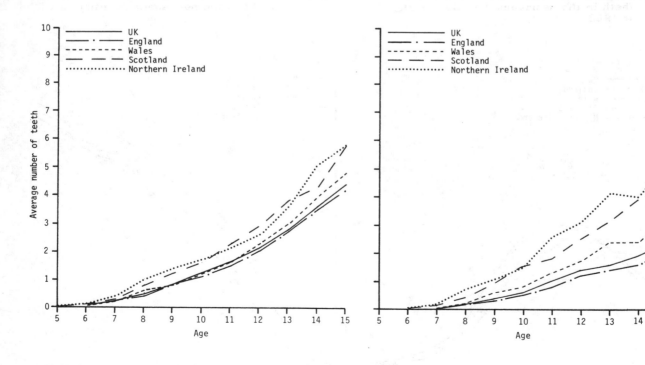

Figure 3.8 shows that there is a considerable variation in the proportion of children with some teeth missing due to decay. Generally, England had the lowest proportion followed in order by Wales, Scotland and Northern Ireland (although among twelve year olds the proportions with some teeth missing due to decay were similar in Scotland and Northern Ireland). The differences between the countries in this proportion were largest among the oldest children. Among fifteen year olds for example, 53% of children from Northern Ireland had at least one tooth missing due to decay, compared with 44% of children from Scotland, 34% of children from Wales and just 21% of children from England.

It was also among the older children that there were the main variations between countries in the average number of permanent teeth missing due to decay (Table 3.2). Overall this average was low, not rising above one tooth in any of the age groups in the United Kingdom as a whole. However, among fourteen year olds, for example, the average number of teeth missing due to decay was twice as high among children in Scotland and Northern Ireland than among children in England or Wales.

Table 3.2   Average number of permanent teeth missing due to decay in the United Kingdom

Age	England	Wales	Scotland	Northern Ireland	United Kingdom
5	—	—	—	—	—
6	—	—	—	—	—
7	—	—	—	—	—
8	—	—	0.1	0.1	—
9	0.1	0.1	0.2	0.2	0.1
10	0.1	0.2	0.3	0.3	0.1
11	0.2	0.3	0.4	0.6	0.2
12	0.3	0.3	0.6	0.7	0.3
13	0.3	0.5	0.7	0.9	0.4
14	0.3	0.5	1.0	1.0	0.4
15	0.5	0.8	1.1	1.3	0.6

For bases see Appendix A

3.5 Known decay experience

In Figure 3.9, we look at the proportion of children who had some active decay in their deciduous dentition and/or some filled (otherwise sound) deciduous teeth. Overall, this proportion rises from 51% of the five year olds in the United Kingdom to 71% of the nine year olds and thereafter decreases as the deciduous teeth are lost. As before, it can be seen that Scotland and Northern Ireland are in the least favourable position and England is the most favourable position. The variation between countries was particularly large among the five year olds. In England, 48% of five year olds had some active decay and/or some filled deciduous teeth. This proportion was 66% among five year olds in Wales and 74% among five year olds in Scotland and in Northern Ireland.

Decay experience of permanent teeth can be measured as a combination of teeth that were decayed, filled or missing due to decay. It can be seen from Figure 3.10 that the proportion of children with some decay experience of their permanent dentition increases with age. Among fifteen year olds in the United Kingdom in 1983, 93% had some decay experience. The figure shows that there were, again, very large differences between the countries, particularly among children aged seven to eleven. Northern Ireland had the highest proportion of children with some decay experience and England the lowest. Scotland had a slightly lower proportion of children with some decay experience in the permanent dentition than Northern Ireland, and children from Wales had a slightly higher proportion than children from England. Among nine year olds for example, 79% from Northern Ireland had some decay experience in their permanent teeth compared with 70% from Scotland, 53% from Wales and 48% from England.

The average number of deciduous teeth that were either decayed or filled are shown in Figure 3.11. It can be seen that there is a large disparity between the countries in this average among the five year olds. Children from England had, on average, 1.6 decayed or filled deciduous teeth, compared with 2.6 among five year olds in Wales, 3.2 in Scotland and 3.7 in Northern Ireland. Thus five year olds from Scotland and Northern Ireland had on average twice as many decayed or filled deciduous teeth as five year olds in England.

There were large differences between the countries in the average number of permanent teeth with some decay experience (Figure 3.12), the largest differences being found among the oldest children. Generally, children from Northern Ireland had similar, but slightly higher average numbers of permanent teeth with known decay experience than children from Scotland. These averages were much lower among children in England and in Wales and, generally, lower among children in England than among children in Wales. For example, the average number of permanent teeth with known decay experience among fifteen year olds was 5.6 in England, 6.7 in Wales, 8.4 in Scotland and 9.2 in Northern Ireland.

3.6 Regional variation in dental health in England

We have seen that, in terms of national variation, England was, in 1983, in the most favourable position in terms of decay experience of children's teeth. However, previous studies have shown that within England there is considerable variation in dental health between different regions, in particular that those who live in the South of the country are in a more advantageous position than those in the North. In Chapter 4 we look at changes that took place in dental health in the regions of England and Wales between 1973 and 1983 using the regional groupings employed in the 1973 analyses. In the table section of this report we present some results for dental health according to a regional grouping of health authorities. In this section we look solely at variation between the South and the rest of England.

Figure 3.9 Proportion of children with some decayed or filled deciduous teeth in UK in 1983

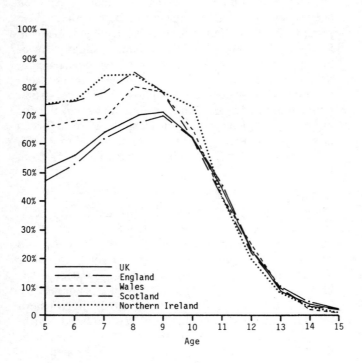

Figure 3.10 Proportion of children with some known decay experience in the permanent dentition in UK in 1983

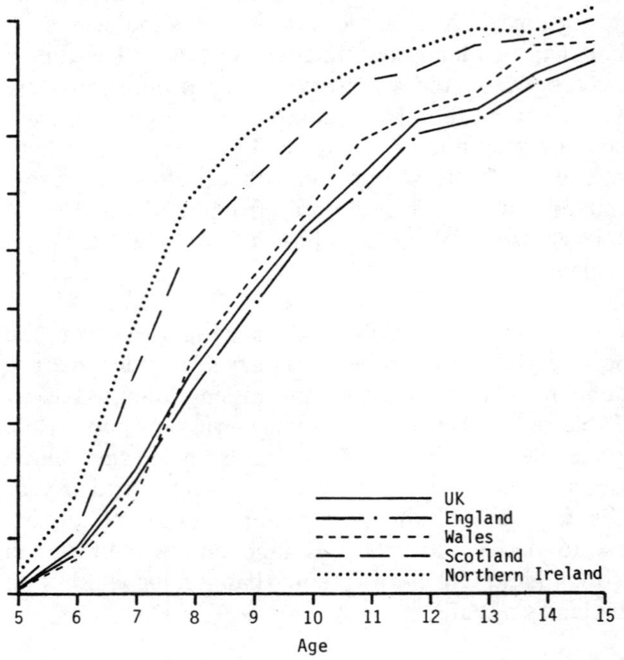

Figure 3.11 Average number of deciduous teeth that were decayed and/or filled in UK in 1983

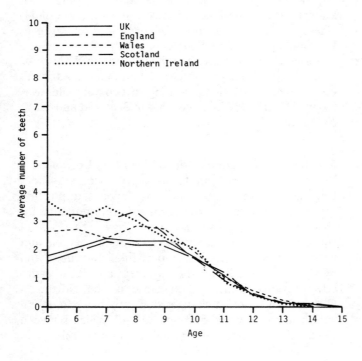

Figure 3.12 Average number of permanent teeth that were decayed, filled and/or missing due to decay in UK in 1983

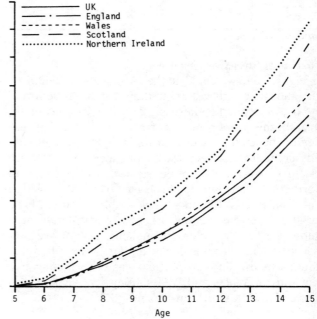

Table 3.3 Average number of deciduous teeth that were decayed or filled for two regional groups in England

Age (years)	The North, the Midlands and East Anglia		The South	
	Average number	Base	Average number	Base
5	1.7	372	1.4	299
6	1.9	388	1.8	329
7	2.4	444	2.1	328
8	2.2	478	2.3	333
9	2.1	542	2.4	349
10	1.8	587	1.7	396
11	1.1	566	1.3	423
12	0.5	552	0.4	419
13	0.1	539	0.2	452
14	0.0	614	0.1	428
15	0.0	577	0.0	400

Table 3.4 Average number of permanent teeth that were decayed, filled or missing (due to decay) for two regional groups in England

Age (years)	The North, the Midlands and East Anglia		The South	
	Average number	Base	Average number	Base
5	0.0	372	0.0	299
6	0.1	388	0.1	329
7	0.4	444	0.2	328
8	0.8	478	0.6	333
9	1.3	542	0.9	349
10	1.8	587	1.3	396
11	2.4	566	2.0	423
12	3.0	552	2.6	419
13	3.9	539	3.3	452
14	4.7	614	4.4	428
15	5.8	577	5.3	400

For this report 'the South' is defined to include the counties of Devon, Cornwall, Somerset, Avon, Dorset, Gloucestershire, Wiltshire, Hampshire, Berkshire, Oxfordshire, Northamptonshire, Buckinghamshire, Bedfordshire, Hertfordshire, Essex, Kent, Sussex, Surrey and Greater London.

Table 3.3 shows that the average number of filled or decayed deciduous teeth is no different among children in the South than among children from the rest of England.

In terms of the average number of permanent teeth that were filled, decayed or missing due to decay, the children from the South were in a better position than children from elsewhere. For example, among thirteen year olds there was an average of 3.3 permanent teeth with known decay experience among children in the South compared with 3.9 teeth among children from the rest of England (Table 3.4). Comparing the rest of England with the other constituent countries of the United Kingdom, children from parts of England other than the South had a lower average number of permanent teeth with known decay experience than children from Wales, Scotland or Northern Ireland.

3.7 The condition of the individual tooth types

Decay does not affect each of the individual tooth types equally. Although disease experience has reduced considerably it is still the case that, in children, the majority of decay is confined to the molars.

Figure 3.13 shows, for children of different ages in the United Kingdom, the condition of certain individual deciduous tooth types. It can be seen that for each of the deciduous incisors, virtually all children had lost them by the age of nine. For the lower incisors only a very small proportion of children had lost their deciduous incisors and had no permanent replacement, but this proportion was slightly higher in the case of upper incisors. A higher proportion of children had decay of their upper incisors than their lower incisors, but in all cases there was very little decay experience found on the deciduous incisors.

There was also very little decay experience on the deciduous canines although a higher proportion of children keep these teeth until past the age of nine than was the case with the deciduous incisors. For example, 52% of ten year olds still retained their upper left canine and the vast majority retained were sound.

A much higher level of decay experience was recorded for the deciduous molars, in particular the second molars. Over a half of the nine year olds retained the upper or lower first deciduous molar. In the case of the lower first deciduous molar a comparatively high proportion of children had lost this tooth but did not yet have the permanent replacement.

In general, the second deciduous molar was retained until an older age than the first molar and was considerably more likely to show evidence of dental disease. For nine year olds, of the upper left second deciduous molars that were examined a quarter were filled and 16% had some active decay. As with the first deciduous molar, a comparatively large proportion of children had lost their lower left second deciduous molar but did not yet have the permanent replacement.

Figure 3.14 shows how individual permanent tooth types were affected by decay. It can be seen that decay experience increased with age but that even among the fifteen year olds less than one in ten of the permanent incisors, canines or first premolars were either decayed or filled. There was a slightly higher proportion of children with decay experience on the second premolars and a higher proportion again with decay experience of the second permanent molars. However, the tooth most likely to have decay experience was the first permanent molar. Among children over the age of eleven, more than a half of their upper and lower left first permanent molars had some decay experience. The major component of this decay experience was evidence of past decay in the form of filled teeth. Among fifteen year olds, for example, the upper left first permanent molar was filled in 57% of cases, extracted, due to decay, in 12% of cases, actively decayed in 9% of cases and sound in just 22% of cases.

Figure 3.13 Decay and treatment experience of individual deciduous teeth

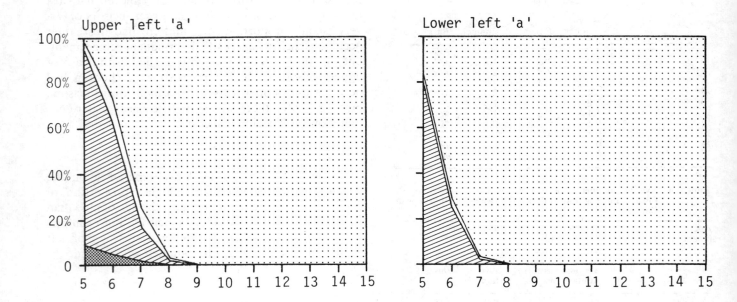

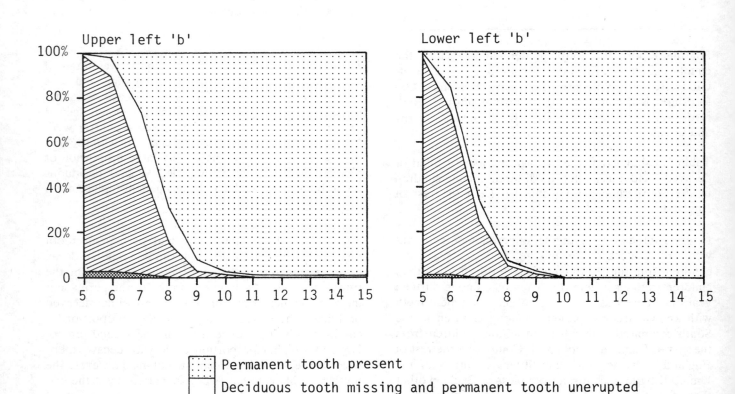

Permanent tooth present
Deciduous tooth missing and permanent tooth unerupted
Sound deciduous tooth
Filled deciduous tooth
Actively decayed deciduous tooth

Figure 3.13 contd

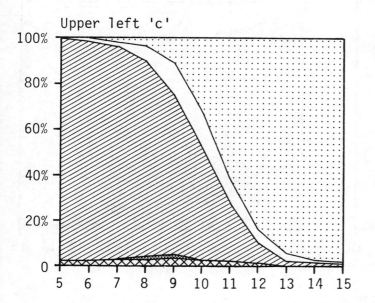

Upper left 'c'

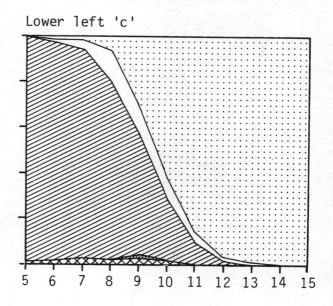

Lower left 'c'

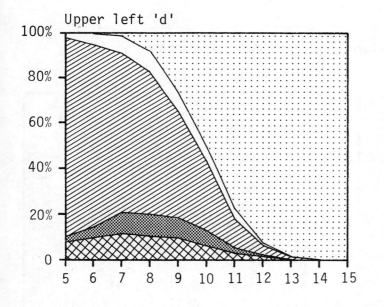

Upper left 'd'

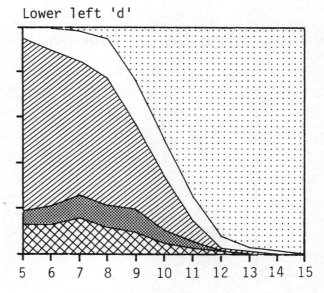

Lower left 'd'

Permanent tooth present
Deciduous tooth missing and permanent tooth unerupted
Sound deciduous tooth
Filled deciduous tooth
Actively decayed deciduous tooth

Figure 3.13 contd

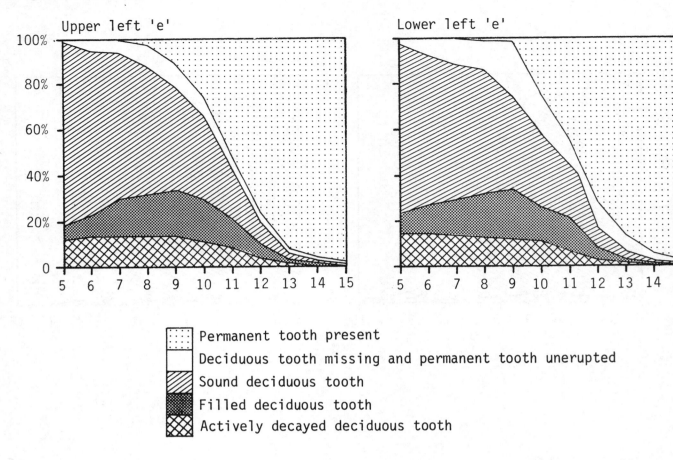

Permanent tooth present

Deciduous tooth missing and permanent tooth unerupted

Sound deciduous tooth

Filled deciduous tooth

Actively decayed deciduous tooth

Figure 3.14 Decay and treatment experience of individual permanent teeth

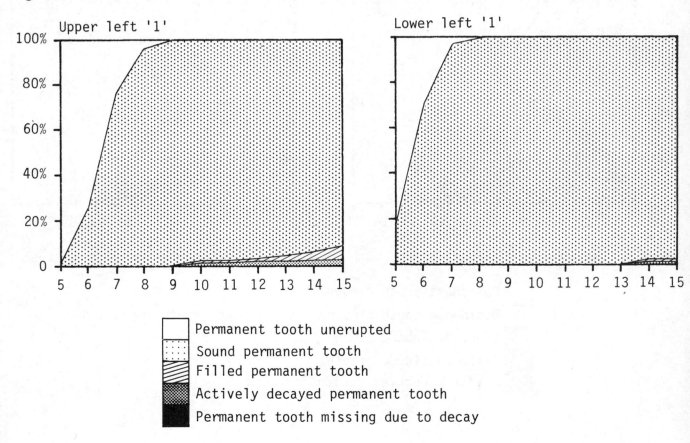

Permanent tooth unerupted

Sound permanent tooth

Filled permanent tooth

Actively decayed permanent tooth

Permanent tooth missing due to decay

Figure 3.14 contd

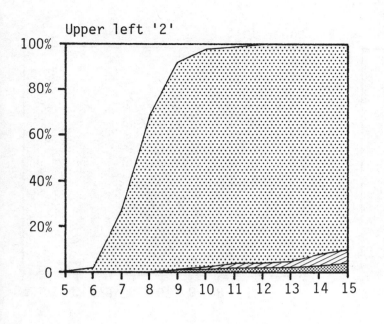

Upper left '2'

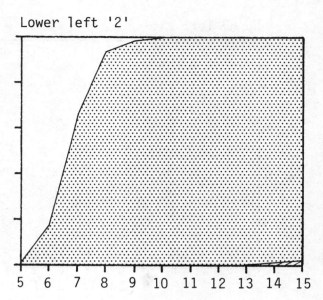

Lower left '2'

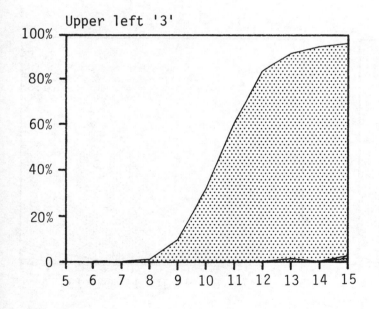

Upper left '3'

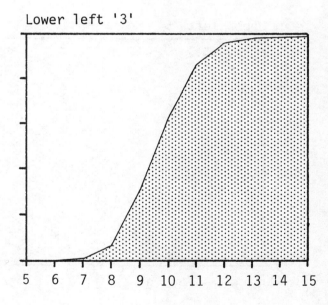

Lower left '3'

Permanent tooth unerupted
Sound permanent tooth
Filled permanent tooth
Actively decayed permanent tooth
Permanent tooth missing due to decay

Figure 3.14 contd

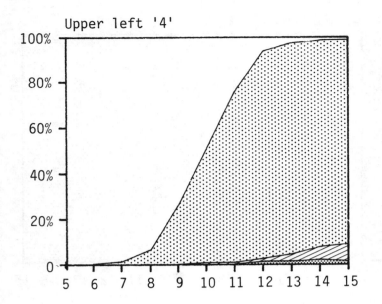

Upper left '4'

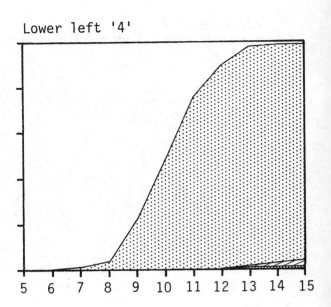

Lower left '4'

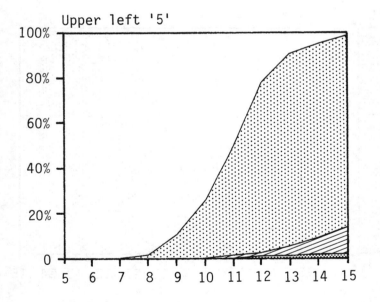

Upper left '5'

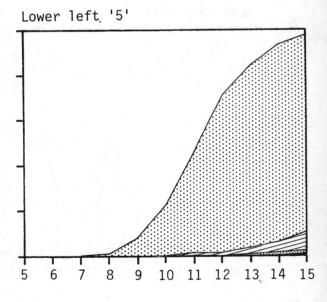

Lower left '5'

☐ Permanent tooth unerupted
⣿ Sound permanent tooth
▨ Filled permanent tooth
▦ Actively decayed permanent tooth
■ Permanent tooth missing due to decay

Figure 3.14 contd

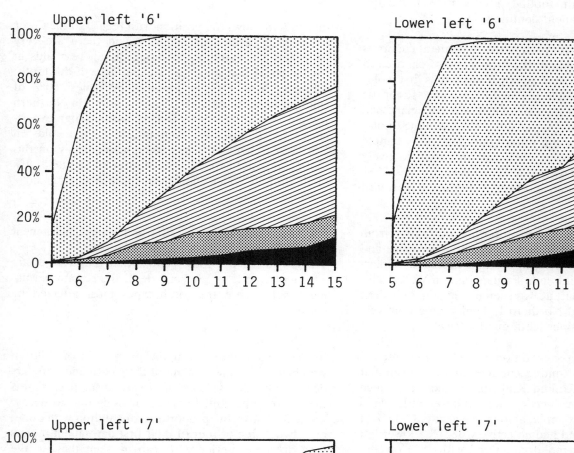

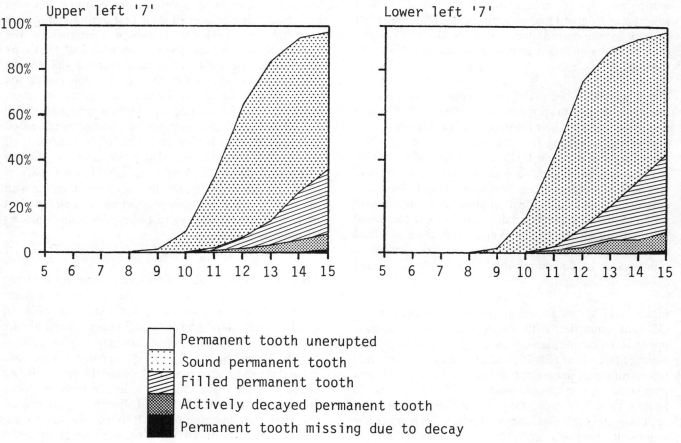

Permanent tooth unerupted
Sound permanent tooth
Filled permanent tooth
Actively decayed permanent tooth
Permanent tooth missing due to decay

3.8 National variation in the condition of individual tooth types

In this section we look at the national variation in the condition of certain tooth types, both from the deciduous and permanent dentition.

Figure 3.15 shows, for each of the constituent countries of the United Kingdom, the proportion of children in each age group who had an upper deciduous first molar that was decayed, filled, sound or missing. It can be seen that a lower proportion of children in England had an actively decayed upper left first deciduous molar than children from the other countries. For example among eight year olds 10% had this tooth actively decayed compared with 16% of children in Wales, 17% of children in Scotland and 16% of children in Northern Ireland.

It can be seen that a higher proportion of children from Scotland and Northern Ireland aged between five and ten no longer had their upper first deciduous molar, compared with children in England and in Wales. This reflects the fact that, as was seen in Chapter 2 children from Scotland and Northern Ireland have a relatively high loss of deciduous teeth due to decay.

Figure 3.16 shows the condition of the lower left second deciduous molars among children in the constituent countries of the United Kingdom. Again, the much lower level of active decay among children in England is apparent. For example, among five year olds, 13% of children in England had an actively decayed lower left second deciduous molar compared with 18% of children in Wales and 28% in both Scotland and Northern Ireland.

There were also very large differences between the countries in the proportions of children of different ages who retained their lower second deciduous molar. For example, among five year olds, 98% of children from England retained this tooth compared with 93% of children from Wales, 88% of children from Scotland and 84% of children from Northern Ireland. Similarly, among eight year olds, 88% of children from England retained their lower second deciduous molar compared with 82% of children from Wales, 68% from Scotland and 65% from Northern Ireland. This again reflects a smaller loss of deciduous teeth due to decay among children in England.

Figure 3.17 shows the proportions of children in the different countries with decay experience on their upper left first permanent molar. It can be seen that among fifteen year olds 76% of children in England had this tooth either decayed, filled or missing due to decay compared with 81% of children in Wales, 90% in Scotland and 92% in Northern Ireland. Proportionately approximately twice as many children in each of the age groups in Scotland and Northern Ireland than in England had lost this tooth due to decay. The figure also shows the particularly high level of active decay on this tooth among children in Northern Ireland. For example among ten year olds in Northern Ireland, 25%

had an actively decayed upper left first permanent molar compared with 16% of children in Scotland, 9% of children in England and 8% of children in Wales.

Figure 3.18 shows the position with regard to the lower left second permanent molar. Again there are very large national variations. Among fifteen year olds in England 41% had some decay experience of this tooth, compared with 50% of children in Wales, 60% of children in Scotland and 71% of children in Northern Ireland. Again, Northern Ireland shows a high experience of active decay. Among fifteen year olds in Northern Ireland 21% had some active decay on this tooth compared with 13% of children in Scotland, 9% of children in Wales and 8% of children in England.

3.9 The condition of the first and second permanent molars

We saw in the previous sections that the first permanent molar and, to a lesser extent, the second permanent molar were the tooth types most affected by decay.

In this section we look at the proportion of children who have all, some or none of their permanent molars decayed or with evidence of disease in the past, that is they were either filled or were missing due to decay. Table 3.5 shows the proportions of children with none, one, two, three or four of their first permanent molars with disease experience. It can be seen that, in the United Kingdom, the proportion who had no decay experience in their first permanent molars decreased with age, and, among fifteen year olds only one in ten children had no decay experience on these teeth. Similarly, the proportion of children who had decay experience on all four first permanent molars increased with age. Among fifteen year olds, 62% had four first permanent molars with decay experience. Among children aged ten and over, it can be seen that, of children with at least one first permanent molar with decay experience, a higher proportion have all four first molars affected than have just one, two or three molars with decay experience.

There was considerable variation in these proportions between the constituents of the United Kingdom. Among fourteen year olds, for example, 50% of children in England had all four first permanent molars with some decay experience, compared with 63% in Wales, 71% in Scotland and 73% in Northern Ireland. Indeed it can be seen that by the time the age of fifteen is reached only one child in a hundred in Northern Ireland was completely free of disease experience on the first permanent molars. It is of interest to see whether the health of the first permanent molar is related to the condition of the other teeth. We examined how many other diseased teeth on average there were per child according to how many first molars a child had that were or had been decayed.

Table 3.5 Distribution of the number of first permanent molars which were decayed, filled, or missing due to decay among children in the United Kingdom

Number of first molars with decay experience	Age (years)										
	5	6	7	8	9	10	11	12	13	14	15
	%	%	%	%	%	%	%	%	%	%	%
England											
0	99	93	81	65	53	39	32	23	20	15	10
1	1	5	8	14	14	16	13	13	10	9	7
2	—	1	6	10	12	14	14	17	12	13	10
3	—	—	3	4	8	11	14	12	16	13	14
4	—	1	2	7	13	20	27	35	42	50	59
Total	100	100	100	100	100	100	100	100	100	100	100
Wales											
0	99	95	85	60	47	35	24	18	16	8	7
1	—	2	8	14	15	15	14	6	7	5	4
2	1	2	4	9	17	22	14	17	11	12	11
3	—	—	1	9	10	8	19	17	15	12	11
4	—	1	2	8	11	20	29	42	51	63	67
Total	100	100	100	100	100	100	100	100	100	100	100
Scotland											
0	98	88	64	39	31	21	14	11	6	5	4
1	1	7	14	16	14	13	9	9	4	4	3
2	1	3	10	16	15	12	13	10	6	9	5
3	—	1	6	12	13	17	17	12	14	11	9
4	—	1	6	17	27	37	47	58	70	71	79
Total	100	100	100	100	100	100	100	100	100	100	100
Northern Ireland											
0	95	84	56	34	22	14	10	7	3	4	1
1	3	7	16	15	11	8	9	5	5	3	2
2	1	6	10	15	14	16	12	10	5	7	6
3	1	1	7	10	17	16	10	16	11	13	9
4	—	2	11	26	36	46	59	62	76	73	83
Total	100	100	100	100	100	100	100	100	100	100	100
United Kingdom											
0	99	92	79	63	50	38	29	21	18	13	9
1	1	5	9	14	14	15	13	12	9	8	6
2	—	2	7	10	13	14	14	16	11	12	10
3	—	—	3	5	9	11	15	13	15	13	13
4	—	1	2	8	14	22	29	38	47	54	62
Total	100	100	100	100	100	100	100	100	100	100	100

For bases see Appendix A

Table 3.6 The average number of permanent teeth with decay experience by the condition of the first molars for children in the United Kingdom

Number of first molars with decay experience	Age (years)																					
	5		6		7		8		9		10		11		12		13		14		15	
0	0.0	*796*	0.0	*794*	0.0	*728*	0.0	*610*	0.0	*530*	0.0	*438*	0.0	*341*	0.1	*245*	0.1	*215*	0.3	*162*	0.4	*104*
1	*	*8*	1.0	*43*	1.0	*83*	1.0	*136*	1.0	*149*	1.0	*173*	1.1	*153*	1.1	*140*	1.3	*107*	1.3	*100*	2.0	*69*
2	–	*0*	*	*17*	2.0	*65*	2.0	*97*	2.0	*138*	2.0	*161*	2.1	*165*	2.3	*186*	2.4	*131*	2.7	*150*	3.0	*116*
3	–	*0*	–	*0*	*	*28*	3.0	*48*	3.1	*95*	3.1	*127*	3.3	*177*	3.4	*151*	3.9	*179*	4.2	*162*	4.5	*150*
4	–	*0*	*	*8*	*	*18*	4.0	*77*	4.2	*149*	4.4	*253*	4.9	*341*	5.5	*443*	6.4	*560*	7.3	*674*	7.9	*717*

* Average numbers not given for bases under 30
  Base figures in italics

Table 3.6 shows the average number of permanent teeth with known decay experience in relation to the number of first molars with decay experience. It can be seen that up to the age of eight, the first molars account for the total disease experience of the permanent teeth and that up to the age of eleven, children with no decayed, filled or missing first molars have no other permanent teeth with decay experience. Decay experience of the permanent teeth increases with age but disproportionately, according to the condition of the first permanent molars, in that children who have a high number of their first molars with disease experience have a higher average of other teeth with disease experience. For example, among fifteen year olds, children with disease-free first permanent molars had an average of 0.4 other teeth with decay experience. Fifteen year olds who had either one or two first molars with decay experience had, on average, one further tooth with decay experience. Fifteen year olds with three first molars with decay experience had, on average, 1.5 further teeth with decay experience while fifteen year olds with all their first molars with decay experience had an average of 3.9 further teeth with decay experience.

Figure 3.15 The condition of the upper left first deciduous molar

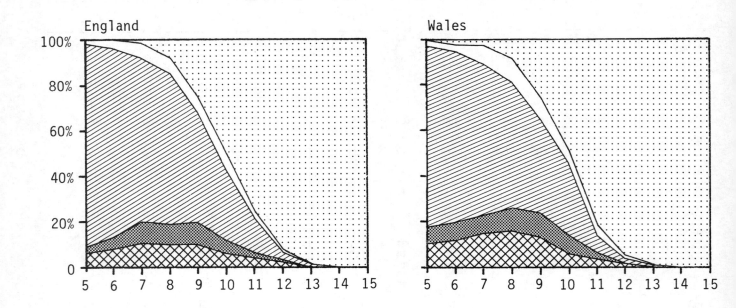

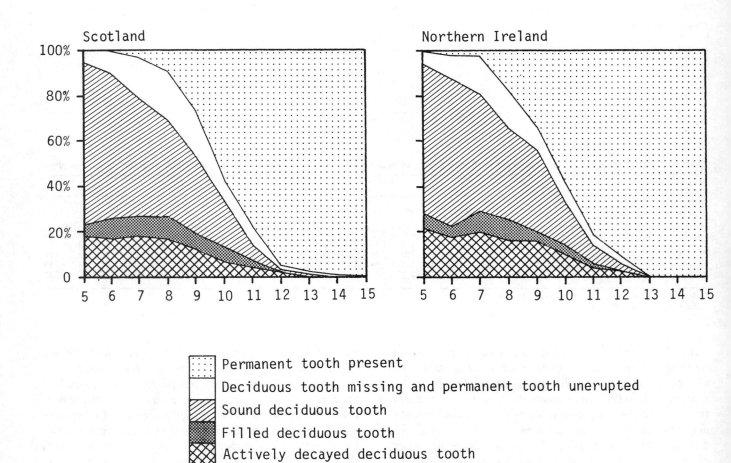

Permanent tooth present
Deciduous tooth missing and permanent tooth unerupted
Sound deciduous tooth
Filled deciduous tooth
Actively decayed deciduous tooth

Figure 3.16 The condition of the lower left second deciduous molar

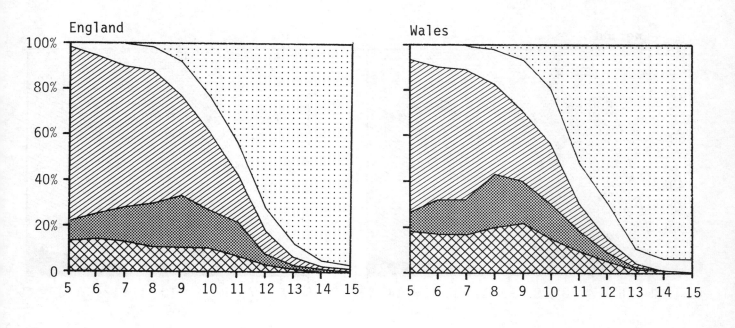

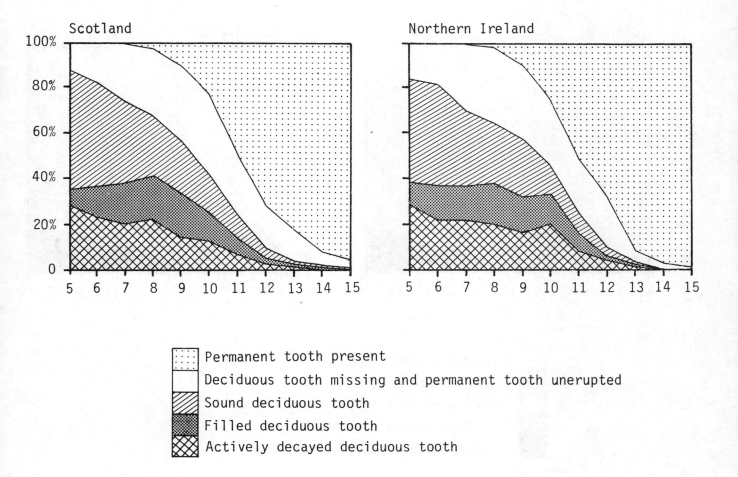

Permanent tooth present

Deciduous tooth missing and permanent tooth unerupted

Sound deciduous tooth

Filled deciduous tooth

Actively decayed deciduous tooth

Figure 3.17 The condition of the upper left first permanent molar

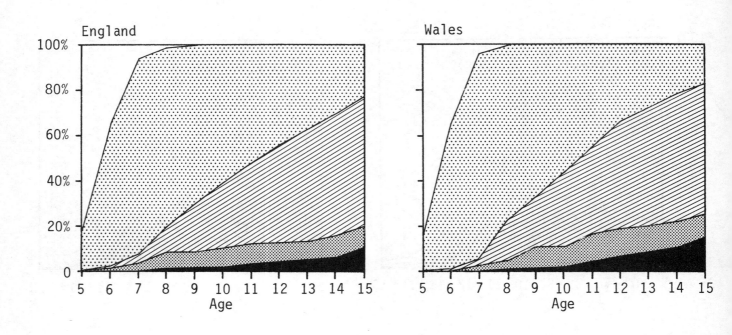

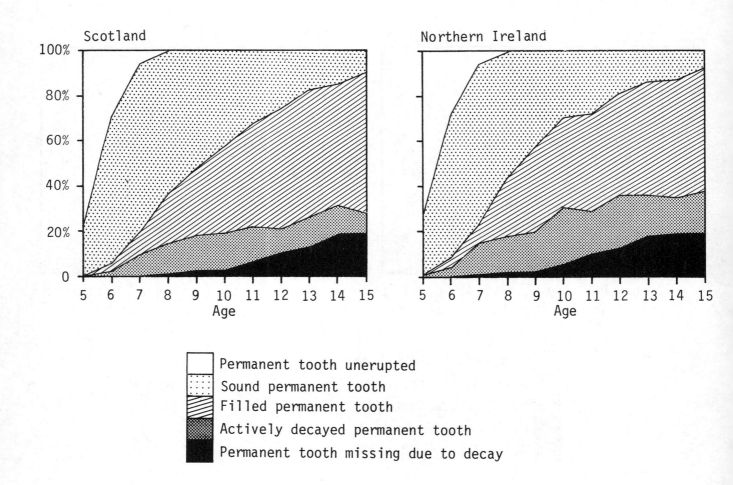

Permanent tooth unerupted
Sound permanent tooth
Filled permanent tooth
Actively decayed permanent tooth
Permanent tooth missing due to decay

Figure 3.18 The condition of the lower left second permanent molar

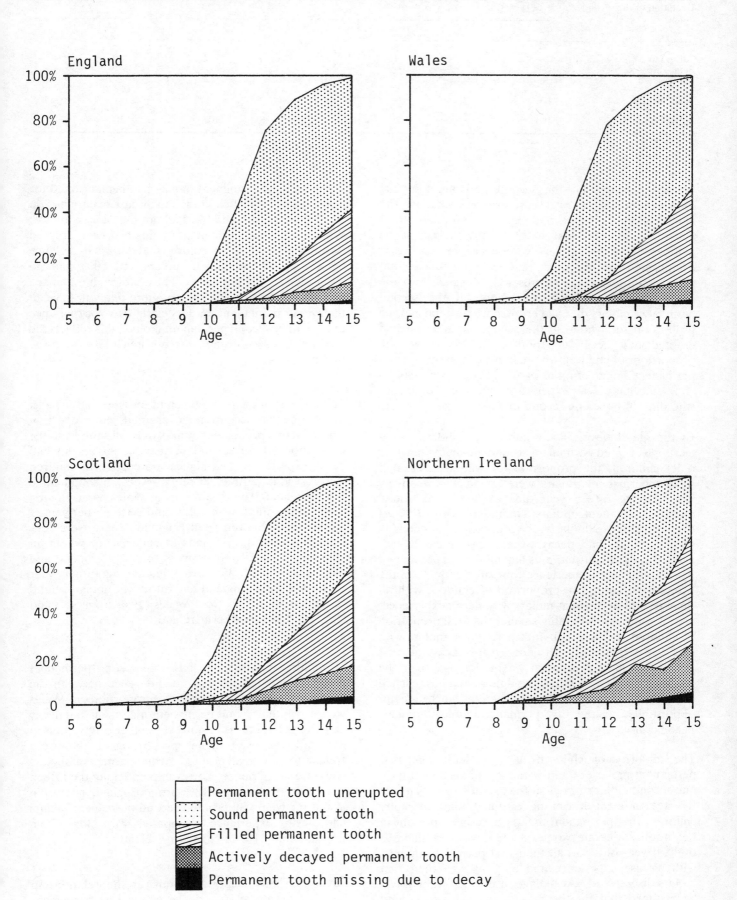

Permanent tooth unerupted
Sound permanent tooth
Filled permanent tooth
Actively decayed permanent tooth
Permanent tooth missing due to decay

Table 3.7   The condition of the second permanent molars among children in the United Kingdom

Condition of the second molar	Age (years)										
	5	6	7	8	9	10	11	12	13	14	15
	%	%	%	%	%	%	%	%	%	%	%
All sound	—	1	1	1	5	20	48	67	63	50	36
Some diseased	—	—	—	—	—	2	5	15	25	36	44
All diseased	—	—	—	—	—	1	2	2	7	13	20
None present	100	99	99	99	95	77	45	16	5	1	—
All second molars	100	100	100	100	100	100	100	100	100	100	100

For bases see Appendix A

We saw earlier that the second permanent molars showed some degree of disease experience among the older children. The second permanent molars erupt much later than the first molars so any analysis of the number of second molars with decay experience is complicated by the fact that not all the second permanent molars may be present. Table 3.7 shows the proportions of children for whom all the second permanent molars that had erupted were sound and the proportion for whom all the second molars that had erupted had decay experience. It also shows the proportions of children who had more than one second permanent molar erupted of which some were sound and some had decay experience, and the proportions who did not have any second molars.

By the age of eleven, about half of the children had at least one erupted permanent second molar. Among the older children, the proportion for whom all erupted second permanent molars were sound was relatively low. Among fifteen year olds, 36% had all sound second permanent molars compared with 67% of twelve year olds. Similarly, the proportion for whom all second molars had decay experience increased with age; 20% of fifteen year olds had all second permanent molars with decay experience compared with 2% of the twelve year olds. The proportion of children with all their second permanent molars with decay experience, was of course considerably smaller than the proportion of children with all their first permanent molars with decay experience. This is not surprising as the first permanent molars erupt at an earlier age than the second molars and thus, by the time a child has reached early teens, there will have been a much greater opportunity for the first permanent molars to have become diseased.

The majority of children have at least one first permanent molar erupted at the age of six and at least one second molar through at the age of eleven. Thus at the age of eight it can be assumed that for many children, first permanent molars have been present in the mouth for about two years and it was seen that 8% of eight year olds had all their first permanent molars with disease experience and 63% had all their first molars disease free. At the age of thirteen when it can be assumed that for the majority of children second molars have been in the mouth for about two years, 7% of children had all their second molars diseased and 63% had them all disease free.

When the first permanent molars had been erupted for three years, 14% of children had disease experience on all of these teeth and 50% had no disease experience. When the second permanent molars had been erupted for three years, 13% of children had disease experience on all second permanent molars and 50% had no disease experience on them. Thus, although on an age by age comparison children are more likely to have all their first permanent molars with decay experience than all their second permanent molars, this reflects the fact that the second molars erupt much later than the first molars.

Table 3.8 shows, for those children who had at least one permanent second molar erupted, the proportion whose second permanent molars were all sound and the proportion whose second permanent molars all had decay experience. The highest proportion of children whose second permanent molars were all sound came from England. The children from Wales had a slightly lower proportion with all sound second permanent molars than children from England. There were considerably lower proportions of children for whom all second permanent molars were sound in Scotland and Northern Ireland. For example, among fifteen year olds, 38% from England had all second molars sound compared with 32% from Wales, 19% from Scotland and 14% from Northern Ireland.

Of children who had at least one second permanent molar erupted, there was no difference between the proportions in England and the proportions in Wales whose erupted second permanent molars all had decay experience. There were however higher proportions in Scotland and even higher proportions in Northern Ireland for whom all erupted second permanent molars had decay experience. For example, among the fifteen year olds, there were 18% from England and from Wales for whom all erupted second permanent molars had decay experience, compared with 30% from Scotland and 41% in Northern Ireland.

Finally, in this section we look at the relationship between the decay experience of the first permanent molars and the decay experience of the second permanent molars. Table 3.9 shows, for all children aged twelve and over with at least one permanent second

Table 3.8 The condition of the second permanent molars among children in the constituent countries of the United Kingdom

Country	Age									
	11		12		13		14		15	
	Of children with at least one second molar, proportion whose second molars were all sound									
England	90%	524	80%	815	69%	941	54%	1,032	38%	967
Wales	83%	177	80%	224	60%	270	48%	261	32%	279
Scotland	79%	297	66%	462	48%	487	37%	582	19%	486
Northern Ireland	79%	144	64%	198	38%	268	34%	225	14%	217
United Kingdom	87%	643	80%	984	66%	1,136	50%	1,237	36%	1,156
	Of children with at least one second molar, proportion whose second molars all had decay experience									
England	2%	524	4%	815	6%	941	11%	1,032	18%	967
Wales	3%	177	1%	224	6%	270	11%	261	18%	279
Scotland	2%	297	7%	462	12%	487	19%	582	30%	486
Northern Ireland	2%	144	7%	198	13%	268	27%	225	41%	217
United Kingdom	3%	643	2%	984	7%	1,136	13%	1,237	20%	1,156

molar erupted, the proportion with disease experience of the second molars, according to how many first molars had disease experience. In each of the age groups, but particularly among the older children, it can be seen that a high proportion of children with no first permanent molars with decay experience, had all sound second permanent molars while a very high proportion of children with four first permanent molars with decay experience, had some decay experience of their second molars. For example, among fifteen year olds with at least one second permanent molar erupted,

80% of those with no decay experience of their first permanent molars had no decay experience on their second molars, while just 20% did have some decay experience on these teeth. For those who had all four diseased first molars, only 22% were completely free of decay experience on their second molars. About a half (48%) of these children had some diseased and some sound second molars while 30% of those who had all their first molars with decay experience also had all their erupted second molars affected by disease.

Table 3.9 The relationship between the decay experience of the first molars and the decay experience of the second molars for children in the United Kingdom with at least one second molar erupted

Second molars	Number of first molars with decay experience				
	0	1	2	3	4
Twelve year olds	%	%	%	%	%
All sound	92	96	89	87	70
Some diseased	8	4	9	11	23
All diseased	—	—	2	2	7
Total	100	100	100	100	100
Base	193	109	156	128	394
Thirteen year olds					
All sound	97	90	82	64	44
Some diseased	2	8	17	32	43
All diseased	1	2	1	4	13
Total	100	100	100	100	100
Base	198	102	123	172	543
Fourteen year olds					
All sound	92	81	71	60	30
Some diseased	8	19	27	37	47
All diseased	—	—	2	3	23
Total	100	100	100	100	100
Base	159	99	148	160	667
Fifteen year olds					
All sound	80	58	55	48	22
Some diseased	19	41	42	46	48
All diseased	1	1	3	6	30
Total	100	100	100	100	100
Base	102	69	116	150	717

Table 3.10   The provision of fissure sealants among children in the United Kingdom

Country	Age (years)										
	5	6	7	8	9	10	11	12	13	14	15
	Proportion of children with some fissure sealants										
England	–	1%	5%	5%	6%	4%	3%	3%	4%	2%	2%
Wales	–	2%	6%	9%	6%	7%	4%	4%	5%	2%	2%
Scotland	2%	8%	12%	18%	13%	14%	16%	13%	13%	12%	7%
Northern Ireland	1%	5%	6%	3%	4%	2%	2%	1%	1%	1%	–
United Kingdom	–	2%	5%	6%	6%	4%	4%	4%	5%	3%	2%

For bases see Appendix A

3.10 Fissure sealants

Fissure sealants are applied to the surfaces of the teeth in order to arrest or prevent dental decay. It was not thought that, in 1983, the provision of fissure sealants would be widespread but it was decided to collect information at the dental examination about children with sealants so that if future national studies were to be carried out there would be a baseline figure for comparison.

Table 3.10 shows the proportions of children with some fissure sealants. In the United Kingdom as a whole, as expected, only a small proportion of children had been provided with fissure sealants. This proportion was highest (6%) among the eight and nine year olds. There are several possible reasons for this slight peak among the middle age group. First, sealants are normally applied to the permanent molars or premolars so they can only be applied after the eruption of these teeth. In addition, sealants are only applied to unfilled surfaces. If the provision of sealants is a fairly recent occurrence then many of the older children may not be able to be provided with them, due to the fact that their molars are already filled or, indeed, lost for decay reasons. Indeed, it was shown earlier that 62% of fifteen year olds in the United Kingdom had all their first molars either decayed, filled or missing due to decay while only 14% of nine year olds had all their first molars affected in this way. One further contributing factor to the slightly lower proportion of older children may be that they had been provided with them when they were younger but that they had since fallen off.

Table 3.10 also shows how the proportion of children with fissure sealants varies between the countries of the United Kingdom. Generally there was little difference between the proportions of children in England, Wales and Northern Ireland with some fissure sealants, although among the eight and ten year olds there was a lower proportion in Northern Ireland, than in Wales, with fissures sealants. There was, however, a considerably higher proportion of children in Scotland who had been provided with fissure sealants. For example, among eight year olds, 18% from Scotland had some fissure sealants compared with 5% among children from England, 9% among children from Wales and 3% among children from Northern Ireland. Among eleven year olds, 16% from Scotland had some fissure sealants compared with 4% among children from England, 3% among children from Wales and 2% among children from Northern Ireland. (A closer investigation of the result from Scotland showed that the random selection of schools included a few where there was a very high percentage of children with fissure sealants and this has contributed to the high overall proportion of children in that country with sealants.)

3.11 Summary

Ideally dental decay should be prevented but once it exists it needs to be treated so that the condition of the tooth does not deteriorate to such an extent that it has to be extracted. The dental examination collected information about the disease experience of the teeth, recording whether active decay was present, restorative work had been carried out or, with respect to the permanent dentition, whether teeth had been extracted due to decay. The results were examined to establish whether there were any differences in known decay experience and the treatment received by children in the constituent countries of the United Kingdom.

With respect to decay experience of the permanent dentition, the average number of teeth that were either decayed, filled or missing due to caries was highest in Northern Ireland, followed by Scotland, Wales and England. The average number of permanent teeth with active decay, and the average number extracted for decay reasons followed the same pattern. The average number of filled permanent teeth was higher in Northern Ireland and Scotland than elsewhere, reflecting their greater level of decay experience.

It was the molars in both deciduous and permanent dentitions which made the greater contribution to the decay experience of children and the condition of particular tooth types varied very markedly in different parts of the United Kingdom.

Among 15 year olds nearly two thirds of children in the United Kingdom had had decay in all four first permanent molars. Those 15 year olds who had no decay experience on their first permanent molars had on average 0.4 other teeth that had had some decay; those who had one or two first molars that were or had been decayed had on average one other tooth affected by decay. Those who had three permanent first molars affected by decay had on average a further 1.5 teeth affected and those who had all four permanent first molars affected by decay had in addition, on average, a further 3.9 teeth affected by decay elsewhere in the mouth.

Since the time of the first national survey of children's teeth in 1973 there has been considerable development in dental techniques and, for example, the application of fissure sealants to arrest or prevent dental decay has been introduced. It was not thought that the provision of fissure sealants would be widespread in 1983 but their presence in the mouth was recorded in the dental examination so that a base line could be established for future monitoring purposes; 6% of 8 year olds and 9 year olds were recorded as having fissure sealants present. Somewhat higher levels were recorded in Scotland due to the inclusion in the random sample of a few schools where there had been high levels of the application of fissure sealants.

Table 3.11 Average number of teeth with known decay experience for children of different ages, in 1983

Age	England	Wales	Scotland	Northern Ireland	United Kingdom	England	Wales	Scotland	Northern Ireland	United Kingdom
	Average number of decayed deciduous teeth (d)					*Average number of decayed permanent teeth (D)*				
5	1.1	1.8	2.6	3.0	1.3	–	–	–	0.1	–
6	1.2	1.7	2.1	2.2	1.3	0.1	0.1	0.1	0.2	0.1
7	1.2	1.4	1.9	2.5	1.3	0.2	0.1	0.4	0.7	0.2
8	1.0	1.5	2.0	1.8	1.2	0.3	0.3	0.6	0.7	0.3
9	1.0	1.4	1.4	1.4	1.1	0.3	0.4	0.7	0.9	0.4
10	0.7	0.9	0.9	1.2	0.8	0.4	0.4	0.8	1.1	0.5
11	0.5	0.5	0.6	0.5	0.5	0.5	0.8	0.9	1.3	0.6
12	0.2	0.3	0.2	0.3	0.2	0.6	0.7	1.1	1.5	0.6
13	0.1	0.1	0.1	0.1	0.1	0.6	0.9	1.3	1.8	0.7
14	–	–	–	–	–	0.8	1.1	1.5	1.7	0.9
15	–	–	–	–	–	0.9	1.2	1.5	2.1	1.0
	Average number of filled deciduous teeth (f)					*Average number of missing permanent teeth (M)*				
5	0.5	0.8	0.6	0.7	0.5	–	–	–	–	–
6	0.7	1.0	1.1	0.8	0.8	–	–	–	–	–
7	1.1	1.0	1.1	1.1	1.1	–	–	–	–	–
8	1.2	1.3	1.3	1.2	1.2	–	–	0.1	0.1	–
9	1.2	1.2	1.1	1.0	1.2	0.1	0.1	0.2	0.2	0.1
10	1.0	1.0	0.7	0.8	1.0	0.1	0.2	0.3	0.3	0.1
11	0.7	0.5	0.4	0.4	0.6	0.2	0.3	0.4	0.6	0.2
12	0.2	0.2	0.2	0.1	0.2	0.3	0.3	0.6	0.7	0.3
13	0.1	0.1	–	–	0.1	0.3	0.5	0.7	0.9	0.4
14	–	–	–	–	–	0.3	0.5	1.0	1.0	0.4
15	–	–	–	–	–	0.5	0.8	1.1	1.3	0.6
	Average decay experience of deciduous teeth (df)					*Average number of filled permanent teeth (F)*				
5	1.6	2.6	3.2	3.7	1.8	–	–	–	–	–
6	1.9	2.7	3.2	3.0	2.1	–	–	0.1	0.1	–
7	2.3	2.4	3.0	3.5	2.4	0.2	0.2	0.3	0.4	0.2
8	2.2	2.8	3.3	3.0	2.3	0.4	0.6	0.8	1.0	0.5
9	2.2	2.7	2.5	2.4	2.3	0.8	0.8	1.2	1.4	0.8
10	1.7	1.9	1.6	2.0	1.7	1.1	1.2	1.6	1.7	1.2
11	1.2	1.0	0.9	0.9	1.1	1.5	1.6	2.3	2.1	1.6
12	0.4	0.5	0.4	0.4	0.4	2.0	2.3	2.9	2.6	2.1
13	0.1	0.2	0.1	0.1	0.1	2.7	3.0	3.8	3.6	2.8
14	0.1	–	–	–	0.1	3.5	4.0	4.3	5.1	3.6
15	–	–	–	–	–	4.2	4.8	5.8	5.8	4.4
						Average decay experience of permanent teeth (DMF)				
5						–	–	–	0.1	–
6						0.1	0.1	0.2	0.3	0.1
7						0.4	0.3	0.8	1.0	0.4
8						0.7	0.9	1.5	1.9	0.8
9						1.2	1.3	2.1	2.5	1.8
10						1.6	1.8	2.7	3.1	1.8
11						2.2	2.6	3.6	3.9	2.4
12						2.9	3.3	4.5	4.8	3.1
13						3.6	4.5	5.9	6.4	3.9
14						4.6	5.6	6.8	7.7	4.9
15						5.6	6.7	8.4	9.2	5.9
	Sample sizes					*Average decay experience of all teeth (DMF + df)*				
5	671	190	319	198	804	1.6	2.6	3.3	3.8	1.8
6	717	211	357	202	863	2.0	2.8	3.4	3.8	2.2
7	772	225	357	201	921	2.7	2.7	3.8	4.6	2.8
8	811	213	412	202	968	2.9	3.7	4.8	4.9	3.2
9	891	262	401	225	1,061	3.4	3.9	4.5	5.0	3.5
10	983	249	416	224	1,152	3.4	3.6	4.3	5.1	3.5
11	989	272	479	233	1,177	3.4	3.7	4.5	4.9	3.5
12	971	258	525	239	1,165	3.3	3.8	4.9	5.2	3.5
13	991	281	507	276	1,192	3.7	4.7	6.0	6.5	4.1
14	1,042	264	588	227	1,248	4.7	5.6	6.8	7.8	5.0
15	967	279	486	217	1,156	5.6	6.7	8.5	9.2	6.0

4 Dental decay and treatment in England and Wales 1973 and 1983

4.1 Introduction

The 1983 survey of children's dental health covered many of the topics that were covered by the 1973 survey of children's dental health which was carried out in England and Wales. For the assessment of the health of the teeth, identical criteria were used in the two surveys and thus direct comparisons can be made between the dental health of children in 1973 and 1983. In the previous chapter, the measure of known decay experience was discussed and used to show how dental health varied between the constituent countries of the United Kingdom. In this chapter, we use this measure of known decay experience, and its component parts (that is, decayed teeth, filled teeth, and teeth extracted due to decay) to look at how the dental health of children has changed in the ten years between 1973 and 1983.

4.2 Active decay

The measure of active decay includes teeth which were currently decayed at the time of the dental examination and thus represent a current treatment need. Included in this category are teeth which are decayed with no evidence of past treatment, teeth which have been treated in the past but are currently in need of treatment and teeth which have decayed to the point where they are unrestorable and consequently in need

of extraction. Figures 4.1 and 4.2 show the proportion of children in 1973 and 1983 who had at least one tooth which was actively decayed shown separately for the deciduous and permanent dentitions.

It is immediately obvious that there is a very much lower proportion of children with some active decay in 1983 than was the case in 1973. In 1973, over a half of the children aged ten or under had some active decay in their deciduous teeth and, similarly, over half of children aged eleven or over had some active decay in their permanent teeth. In 1983, it can be seen that in all age groups, less than half of the children had any active decay in either their deciduous or permanent teeth. Among five year olds, the proportion with some active decay in their deciduous teeth was 63% in 1973 compared to 38% in 1983 and among eight year olds the level fell from 72% in 1973 to 47% in 1983. There were similarly large decreases found in active decay of the permanent dentition. For example, among eight year olds, the proportion with some active decay in their permanent dentition more than halved, decreasing from 40% in 1973 to 17% in 1983. Among fourteen year olds, the proportion had decreased from 61% in 1973 to 37% in 1983, a drop of 24 percentage points.

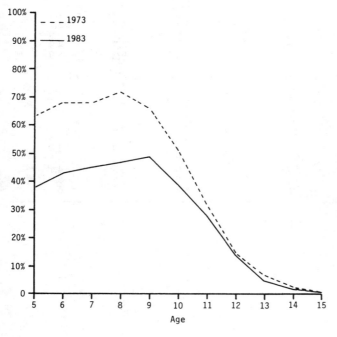

Figure 4.1 Proportion of children with some decayed deciduous teeth in England and Wales in 1973 and 1983

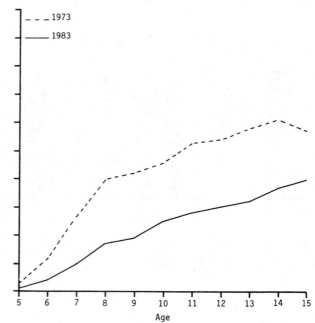

Figure 4.2 Proportion of children with some decayed permanent teeth in England and Wales in 1973 and 1983

Figure 4.3 Average number of decayed deciduous teeth in England and Wales in 1973 and 1983

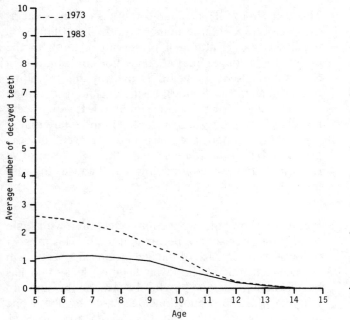

Figure 4.4 Average number of decayed permanent teeth in England and Wales in 1973 and 1983

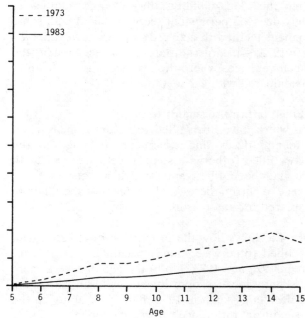

Figures 4.3 and 4.4 show the average number of teeth with active decay per child in 1973 and 1983 for the deciduous and permanent dentitions. In the age range five to seven, children had on average one less deciduous tooth with active decay in 1983 than in 1973. For example, among six year olds, there was an average of 2.5 actively decayed deciduous teeth in 1973 compared with an average of 1.0 in 1983. In the age range seven to fourteen the average number of permanent teeth with active decay had halved between 1973 and 1983. For example, among thirteen year olds this average had decreased from 1.6 in 1973 to 0.7 in 1983.

Of course, if, as we have seen, the proportion of children with some active decay has decreased between the two surveys, it is not surprising that the average number of teeth affected has also decreased. It is of interest to see whether, among those children who had some actively decayed teeth, the average number of

affected teeth had decreased (Table 4.1). Because, as has been shown, the proportion of children with some active decay was so much lower in 1983 than in 1973 the number of children in each of the age groups in Table 4.1 is smaller for the 1983 sample than for the 1973 sample.

Among the younger children it can be seen that the average number of actively decayed deciduous teeth per child with some active decay was lower in 1983 than in 1973. Among five year olds, for example, this average was 4.9 in 1973 compared with 2.9 in 1983. There was no difference in this average among the older children.

Looking at the permanent dentition, there was no statistically significant difference between the average number of actively decayed permanent teeth per child with some actively decayed permanent teeth in 1973 and 1983 among the younger age groups. (The appa-

Table 4.1   Average number of actively decayed teeth among children in England and Wales with some active decay in 1973 and 1983

Age (years)	Deciduous teeth				Permanent teeth			
	1973		1983		1973		1983	
	Average number	*Base*	Average number	*Base*	Average number	*Base*	Average number	*Base*
5	4.1	*600*	2.9	*273*	*	*29*	*	*7*
6	3.7	*734*	2.8	*331*	1.7	*130*	2.5	*31*
7	3.4	*773*	2.7	*373*	1.9	*307*	2.0	*83*
8	2.8	*786*	2.3	*407*	2.0	*436*	1.8	*147*
9	2.4	*745*	2.0	*469*	1.9	*459*	1.6	*182*
10	2.4	*557*	1.8	*408*	2.2	*502*	1.6	*262*
11	1.9	*316*	1.8	*296*	2.5	*523*	1.8	*296*
12	1.3	*143*	1.4	*145*	2.6	*516*	2.0	*311*
13	1.4	*64*	2.0	*53*	2.8	*531*	2.2	*340*
14	*	*18*	*	*22*	3.1	*563*	2.2	*410*
15	*	*7*	*	*20*	2.8	*397*	2.3	*415*

* Average numbers not given for bases under 30.

rent increase in this average among the six year olds is not in fact statistically significant as it was based on so few children, because so few young children in 1983 had any permanent teeth that were actively decayed.)

Among the older children, the average number of actively decayed permanent teeth per child with some permanent teeth with active decay was lower in 1983 than in 1973. The largest difference was seen among the fourteen year olds where the average was 3.1 teeth in 1973 compared with 2.2 teeth in 1983.

4.3 Filled (otherwise sound) teeth
Teeth which have been filled represent a measure of past dental decay and treatment. Included in the category filled (otherwise sound) teeth were all teeth which had been filled and on which there was no evidence of current decay and no need for the filling to be replaced for any reason.

Figure 4.5 shows how the proportion of children with some filled (otherwise sound) deciduous teeth varies between 1973 and 1983. Up to the age of seven, there were slightly lower proportions of children with some filled deciduous teeth in 1983 than 1973, although the only significant difference was seen among the six year olds where the proportion decreased from 38% to 30%. From the age of eight upwards, however, there were

higher proportions of children with some filled deciduous teeth in 1983 than in 1973; among the ten years olds the proportion had increased from 33% of the children in 1973 to 44% in 1983.

The decision to fill a deciduous tooth is not the same as the decision to fill a permanent tooth. The filling of a deciduous tooth, although preserving a tooth in the mouth for a longer period, does not contribute to a child's ultimate dental health in the way that the filling of a permanent tooth does, as the deciduous dentition will naturally exfoliate during childhood. It would seem however from the results presented in the figure that in 1983 more importance was being placed on the preservation of deciduous teeth through restorative treatment among the older children, than was the case in 1973.

Figure 4.6 shows the proportions of children with some filled (otherwise sound) permanent teeth. This proportion was lower in each of the age groups in 1983 than in 1973, which reflects the lower level of decay that has been commented upon previously. Among the nine and ten year olds the proportions decreased by about one quarter between 1973 and 1983, from 50% to 36% among the nine year olds and from 61% to 46% among the ten year olds.

Figure 4.5 Proportion of children with some filled deciduous teeth in England and Wales in 1973 and 1983

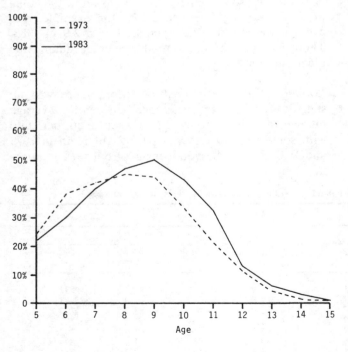

Figure 4.6 Proportion of children with some filled permanent teeth in England and Wales in 1973 and 1983

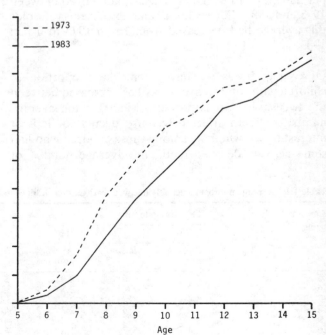

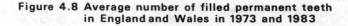

Figure 4.7 Average number of filled deciduous teeth in England and Wales in 1973 and 1983

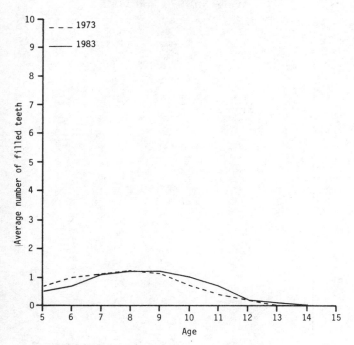

Figure 4.8 Average number of filled permanent teeth in England and Wales in 1973 and 1983

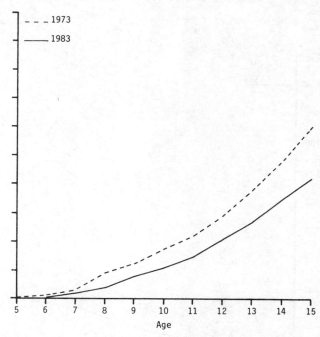

Figures 4.7 and 4.8 show how the average number of filled teeth per child has changed over the last ten years. There was in fact no statistically significant difference between the average number of filled deciduous teeth in 1973 and 1983 but there was a statistically significant decrease in the average number of permanent filled teeth. This decrease was particularly large among the oldest children where, for example, among fifteen year olds the average number of filled permanent teeth decreased from 6.0 in 1973 to 4.2 in 1983. Table 4.2 shows that the results are similar if one looks at the average number of filled teeth among children who had some fillings. There was little difference between 1973 and 1983 among the deciduous teeth, but among permanent teeth there was a decrease in the number of filled teeth, with, for example, the average number of filled teeth per fifteen year old with any fillings decreasing by 1.9 teeth.

4.4 Permanent teeth missing due to decay

Teeth which are currently decayed represent a situation of current treatment need while teeth which are filled and sound represent past treatment. Permanent teeth

that have been lost due to decay also measure the level of past decay. These teeth represent an irreversible situation in that, of course, these teeth cannot be replaced. In this section we look at how the situation with regard to these missing teeth has changed over the ten years between surveys. In the previous two sections we have looked at measures of dental health as they affected both the deciduous and permanent teeth but, as was discussed in Chapter 2, an assessment was not made, by the dentist at the time of the examination, of the reason for loss of the deciduous teeth. In Chapter 2 various assumptions were made about the reasons for loss of deciduous teeth, and figures were presented comparing estimates of the total decay experience of the deciduous dentition made under these assumptions in 1983 with estimates made under similar assumptions in 1973. Whichever assumption was taken, it was shown that among five year olds the total decay experience of the deciduous teeth was much lower in 1983 than in 1973; under the most realistic assumption, the average number of deciduous teeth with decay experience had decreased from 4.0 teeth in 1973 to 1.8 teeth in 1983.

Table 4.2 Average number of filled teeth among children in England and Wales with some filled teeth in 1973 and 1983

Age (years)	Deciduous teeth				Permanent teeth			
	1973		1983		1973		1983	
	Average number	Base	Average number	Base	Average number	Base	Average number	Base
5	2.7	248	2.2	165	*	–	*	–
6	2.6	410	2.3	231	2.0	54	*	23
7	2.6	478	2.8	332	1.8	193	2.0	83
8	2.7	491	2.6	407	2.4	404	1.7	199
9	2.5	497	2.4	478	2.4	564	2.2	311
10	2.1	360	2.3	450	2.8	666	2.4	481
11	1.9	207	2.2	339	3.3	651	2.7	592
12	2.0	96	1.5	135	3.9	717	3.1	704
13	0.0	37	1.7	64	4.9	705	3.8	754
14	*	9	0.0	33	5.9	748	4.4	876
15	*	7	*	10	6.8	612	4.9	882

* Average numbers not given for bases of under 30

Figure 4.9 Proportion of children with some permanent teeth missing due to decay in England and Wales in 1973 and 1983

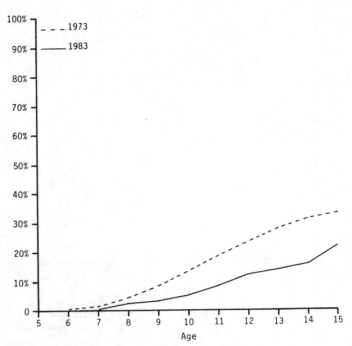

Figure 4.10 Average number of permanent teeth missing due to decay in England and Wales in 1973 and 1983

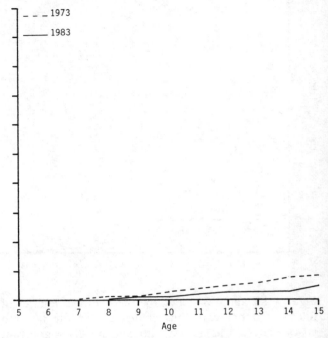

Figure 4.9 shows the proportions of children with some permanent teeth missing due to decay in 1973 and 1983. It can be seen that there was a very significant decrease in this proportion between the two surveys and that in each age group the proportion has decreased by a third or more. Among thirteen year olds, for example, the proportion had halved, from 28% in 1973 to 14% in 1983.

The average number of teeth per child missing due to decay had, in 1973, not been very large and thus the scope for improvement in 1983 was small. However, it can be seen from Figure 4.10 that there had been a small decrease over each of the ages above nine in this average between the two surveys. Table 4.3 shows, however, that if one looks only at the children who had lost some permanent teeth due to decay, the average number of teeth they had lost was no different in 1983 from 1973. (The table only shows figures for children aged ten or more, because so few younger children had lost any permanent teeth.) Thus, it seems that a much higher proportion of children are avoiding the loss of any permanent teeth but that those who do lose teeth due to decay are in a similar position to their counterparts ten years ago.

4.5 Decay experience

We have looked previously at three measures of dental disease experience – actively decayed teeth, filled teeth and teeth extracted due to decay. In this section we combine these measures to present the decay experience of both the deciduous and the permanent dentition.

We have already shown in Chapter 2 that the total decay experience of deciduous teeth has decreased and

because of the difficulties of assessing the reason for loss of these teeth we look in this chapter at the changes that have taken place in the health of the deciduous dentition, in terms of teeth which are actively decayed or which have been filled.

Table 4.3 Average number of teeth missing due to decay among some children in England and Wales with some teeth missing due to decay in 1973 and 1983

Age (years)	Teeth missing			
	1973		1983	
	Average number	Base	Average number	Base
10	2.3	142	2.0	52
11	2.2	177	2.5	85
12	2.2	220	2.5	124
13	2.1	256	2.1	149
14	2.6	286	1.9	177
15	2.4	230	2.3	228

Figure 4.11 shows that the proportion of children with some actively decayed deciduous teeth and/or some filled deciduous teeth was considerably lower in 1983 than in 1973.

Among five year olds, for example, the proportion had decreased by one third from 71% to 48%, that is from almost three quarters of five year olds to one half. We have seen from earlier results that this decrease is due overwhelmingly to the decrease in the proportion of children with actively decayed teeth, rather than a decrease in the proportion with filled teeth.

We define permanent teeth with known decay experience as permanent teeth which were currently decayed, or were filled or which were extracted due to decay.

Figure 4.11 Proportion of children with some filled or decayed deciduous teeth in England and Wales in 1973 and 1983

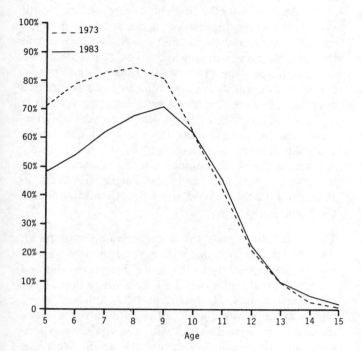

Figure 4.12 Proportion of children with known decay experience of permanent teeth in England and Wales in 1973 and 1983

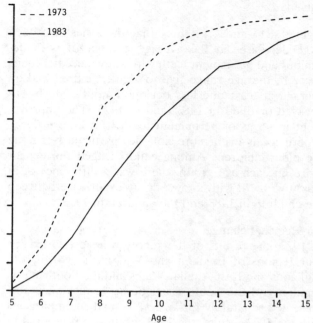

Figure 4.13 Average number of filled or decayed deciduous teeth in England and Wales in 1973 and 1983

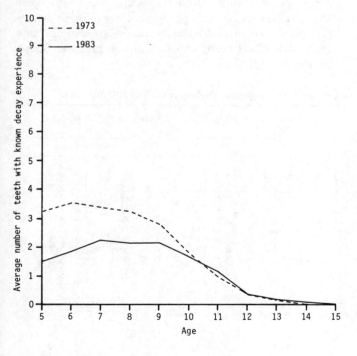

Figure 4.14 Average number of permanent teeth with known decay experience in England and Wales in 1973 and 1983

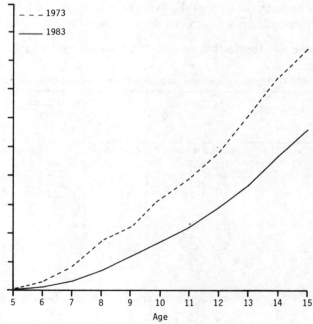

Figure 4.12 shows that the proportion of children with some known decay experience of the permanent dentition was much lower in 1983 than it had been in 1973, particularly among the younger children where in the age range five to eight the proportion had almost halved.

Figures 4.13 and 4.14 show that there has also been large decreases in the average number of both deciduous and permanent teeth with known decay experience. In the age range five to eight, children had on average at least one less deciduous tooth which was decayed or filled in 1983 than in 1973. The improvement in terms of permanent teeth with known decay experience is even more notable, particularly among the older children. Among children aged thirteen or more, in each age group, there was a difference of at least two teeth with known decay experience between the children in 1983 and the children in 1973.

4.6 Regional change

In 1973, the results of the survey were presented for four regions of England and Wales: the North, the Midlands and East Anglia, Wales and the South West, London and the South East. Some results were also presented separately for Wales. To make comparisons with the 1973 results, the 1983 results are presented in this section grouped into the 1973 regions. (In fact, this section deals only with the four regional groupings in England and Wales; a separate chapter presents results for Wales for various aspects of dental health in 1973 and 1983.)

In the previous sections we looked at the various components of known decay experience. In this section, in order to see how dental health has changed in the regions, we look at the average number of teeth in both dentitions with known decay experience.

Table 4.4 shows that among the younger children in each of the regions there was a lower average number of decayed or filled deciduous teeth in 1983 than in 1973. Among five year olds, for example, there had been a reduction in this average in each of the regions of 1.5 deciduous teeth. In 1973, Wales and the South West had had the highest average number of decayed and filled deciduous teeth and generally this was still true in 1983 except among the seven year olds where those children from the North showed the highest average. Generally, among children aged seven and over those from the North showed less improvement in the average number of filled and decayed deciduous teeth than the other regions. For example among seven year olds this average decreased by 0.3 teeth among children in the North, compared with a reduction of 1.5 teeth in the Midlands and East Anglia, 1.6 teeth in Wales and the South West and 1.3 teeth in London and the South East.

The table also shows the average number of filled, decayed and missing (due to decay) permanent teeth in the regions in 1973 and 1983. In 1973, again Wales and the South West had shown a higher average than any of the other regions. However, in 1983, although there had been improvements in all regions in the average number of permanent teeth with known decay experience, the average in Wales and the South West was similar to the average in the North, and both these regions showed a higher average decay experience of the permanent teeth than the Midlands and East Anglia and London and the South East. In 1983, the largest differences between the regions was among the oldest children. Among fifteen year olds those from the North had an average of 6.3 permanent teeth with decay experience and those from Wales and the South West had an average of 6.5 permanent teeth with decay experience. In the Midlands and East Anglia this average was 4.9 teeth and in London and the South East it was 5.1 teeth.

Table 4.4   The average number of teeth with known decay experience among children in the regions of England and Wales 1973 and 1983

Age	The North		The Midlands and East Anglia		Wales and South West		London and South East	
	1973	1983	1973	1983	1973	1983	1973	1983
Average number of decayed and filled deciduous teeth								
5	3.2 *323*	1.7 *221*	3.5 *200*	1.7 *151*	3.7 *158*	2.2 *102*	3.1 *271*	1.5 *245*
6	3.4 *347*	2.1 *232*	3.1 *224*	1.8 *156*	4.1 *168*	2.5 *105*	3.8 *341*	1.8 *277*
7	3.1 *390*	2.8 *245*	3.5 *221*	2.0 *199*	4.0 *185*	2.4 *126*	3.4 *341*	2.1 *259*
8	3.0 *357*	2.3 *260*	3.0 *224*	2.0 *218*	3.8 *166*	2.7 *113*	3.5 *344*	2.2 *274*
9	2.4 *358*	2.2 *323*	2.5 *223*	1.8 *219*	3.2 *169*	2.6 *140*	3.0 *379*	2.4 *275*
10	1.8 *362*	1.8 *328*	1.5 *213*	1.7 *259*	2.3 *163*	1.9 *134*	2.1 *354*	1.7 *325*
11	0.9 *317*	1.0 *327*	1.0 *195*	1.2 *239*	0.9 *155*	1.1 *147*	1.2 *319*	1.3 *345*
12	0.3 *294*	0.5 *319*	0.5 *182*	0.4 *233*	0.6 *160*	0.5 *143*	0.4 *320*	0.4 *341*
13	0.1 *285*	0.1 *308*	0.2 *194*	0.1 *231*	0.1 *146*	0.2 *157*	0.2 *290*	0.2 *366*
14	– *308*	– *356*	0.1 *207*	0.1 *258*	– *145*	0.1 *151*	– *263*	0.1 *344*
15	– *318*	– *334*	0.1 *130*	– *233*	– *111*	– *151*	– *237*	– *320*
Average number of decayed, filled and missing (due to decay) permanent teeth								
5	– *323*	– *221*	– *200*	– *151*	– *158*	– *102*	– *271*	– *245*
6	0.3 *347*	0.2 *232*	0.3 *224*	0.1 *156*	0.3 *168*	0.1 *105*	0.3 *341*	0.1 *277*
7	0.9 *390*	0.6 *245*	0.9 *221*	0.3 *199*	1.0 *185*	0.3 *126*	0.8 *341*	0.2 *259*
8	1.9 *357*	0.9 *260*	1.7 *224*	0.7 *218*	1.7 *166*	0.8 *113*	1.6 *344*	0.6 *274*
9	2.3 *358*	1.4 *323*	2.1 *223*	1.2 *219*	2.4 *169*	1.2 *140*	2.2 *379*	1.0 *275*
10	3.0 *362*	2.0 *328*	3.0 *213*	1.7 *259*	3.1 *163*	1.7 *134*	2.9 *354*	1.3 *325*
11	3.9 *317*	2.5 *327*	3.7 *195*	2.2 *239*	4.4 *155*	2.6 *147*	3.8 *319*	1.9 *345*
12	4.6 *294*	3.3 *319*	4.9 *182*	2.6 *233*	5.0 *160*	3.2 *143*	4.8 *320*	2.6 *341*
13	6.4 *285*	4.2 *308*	5.7 *194*	3.5 *231*	6.7 *146*	4.2 *157*	5.8 *290*	3.3 *366*
14	7.3 *308*	5.0 *356*	6.9 *207*	4.4 *258*	8.5 *145*	5.2 *151*	7.2 *263*	4.4 *344*
15	8.6 *318*	6.3 *334*	8.4 *130*	4.9 *233*	8.8 *111*	6.5 *151*	8.1 *237*	5.1 *320*

Figure 4.15 The condition of the upper left deciduous central incisor

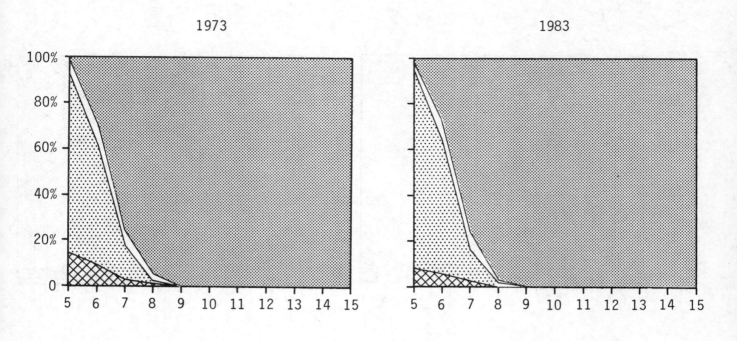

1973

1983

Figure 4.16 The condition of the lower left deciduous first molar

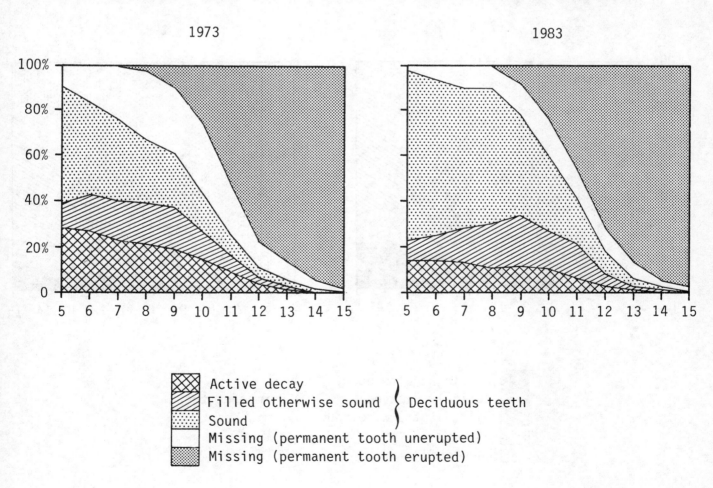

1973

1983

Active decay
Filled otherwise sound } Deciduous teeth
Sound
Missing (permanent tooth unerupted)
Missing (permanent tooth erupted)

Figure 4.17 The condition of the upper left permanent central incisor

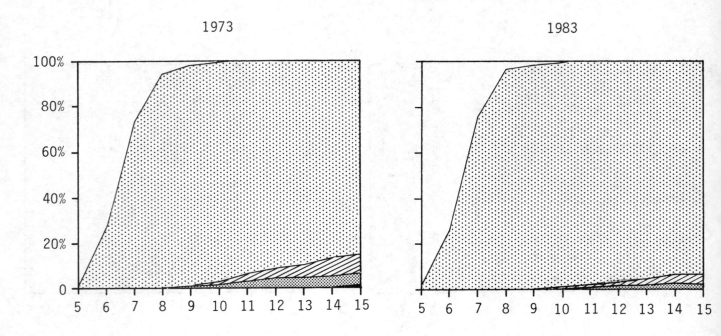

1973

1983

Figure 4.18 The condition of the lower left permanent first molar

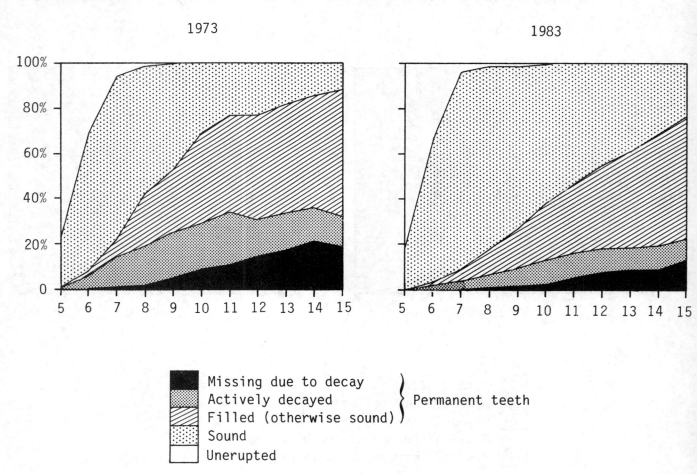

1973

1983

Missing due to decay
Actively decayed   } Permanent teeth
Filled (otherwise sound)
Sound
Unerupted

Generally, among the older children the least improvements were seen in the North. For example among twelve year olds the average number of permanent teeth with decay experience decreased by 1.3 teeth among children in the North compared with 2.3 teeth among children from the Midlands and East Anglia, 1.8 teeth among children from Wales and the South West and 2.2 teeth among children from London and the South East.

4.7 Individual tooth types

So far in this chapter we have looked at the changes in the overall levels of decay experience among children that occurred between 1973 and 1983. In this section we look at changes in the disease pattern of individual tooth types.

Figures 4.15 and 4.16 show the condition of two deciduous tooth types—an incisor and a molar. It can be seen that in both 1973 and 1983 the upper left central incisor was not prone to dental decay (Figure 4.15) but that there had still been a decrease in the proportion that were actively decayed over a period of ten years. For example, in 1973, 15% of five year olds had an actively decayed upper left central deciduous incisor compared with 7% of five year olds in 1983. The overall decrease in active decay in deciduous teeth is also very noticeable on the lower left second deciduous molar (Figure 4.16). Among five year olds the proportion with actively decayed lower left second deciduous molars decreased from 28% in 1973 to 13% in 1983. It is also interesting to see that the proportion of deciduous lower left second molars present in the mouth had increased between 1973 and 1983. The proportion of children who had lost this tooth and did not yet have the permanent replacement was higher in 1973 than was the case in 1983. This is very likely to be due to the fact that a much higher proportion of these teeth would have been lost for decay reasons in 1973 than in 1983.

Figures 4.17 and 4.18 show the decay experience of the upper left permanent central incisor and the lower left permanent first molar. Again it can be seen that, although the incisor shows little disease experience in 1973 this has still decreased by 1983. The change in the condition of the molar, however, is very striking, with large decreases in the proportion of children with decay experience in that tooth. For example among fourteen year olds, 21% had lost this tooth due to decay in 1973 compared with just 8% in 1983. The proportion of children with an actively decayed lower left first molar among the eleven year olds had decreased from 23% in 1973 to 11% in 1983.

4.8 Summary

The purpose of the 1983 survey was to establish the level of dental health among children aged 5 to 15 in the United Kingdom, and to compare for England and Wales the dental health of children in 1973 with the position in 1983. The proportion of children with known decay experience in 1983 was significantly lower than the proportion in 1973. This was so for both dentitions and all ages, although the biggest differences were to be found for 5 year olds and the smallest for 15 year olds. The proportion of children with active decay had declined as had the average number of decayed teeth among children who had some active decay. There were proportionately fewer young children with filled deciduous teeth in 1983 compared with 1973, but more older children with filled deciduous teeth in the later survey. This reflects reduction of disease levels in the younger children and a greater proportion of restored deciduous teeth among those that were diseased in the older children. There were fewer children with any filled permanent teeth in 1983 than had been the case ten years earlier and, as with the deciduous dentition, fewer teeth were recorded as in need of restorative treatment, but the proportion of diseased teeth that had been restored was greater than in 1973.

5 Decay experience in the United Kingdom: the home background

5.1 Introduction

In the previous two chapters it has been shown that the decay experience of children varied considerably between the constituent countries of the United Kingdom but that, in England and Wales, there had been a significant improvement in the condition of children's teeth. These results were based on information collected from all children at the dental examination. In this chapter we look in more detail at the variations in dental decay experience in the United Kingdom by linking the information collected via the dental examination with information collected from the parents via the postal questionnaire.

Questionnaires were sent by post to parents of the children in the sample aged five, eight, twelve and fifteen. Information was collected concerning the child's dental history, in terms of whether they had visited the dentist and what type of treatment they had received; the parents' attitudes towards dental health and their child's teeth; current dental practices such as teeth cleaning and visiting the dentist; and background characteristics of the parents in terms of their dental status and social class. The child's dental history and parental attitudes towards dental health are discussed in a separate chapter. Here, we look at how a child's background is related to his or her dental disease experience.

5.2 Household social class

On the questionnaire that was sent to the children's parents, both parents were asked to record their current or last occupation and from this information their social class was derived. Table 5.1 shows the distribution of children according to their household social class, which was defined as the father's social class unless the father was not in the household, in which case it was the mother's social class. Although, as we have seen, the response rate to the postal survey of parents was very good, some parents were unwilling to provide information concerning their occupation. It can be seen from the table that, in the United Kingdom, between 7% and 10% of parents did not provide us with the necessary information to code social class.

In the United Kingdom as a whole, 43% of five year olds were in Social Classes I, II and III non-manual (IIIN), 36% were in Social Class III manual (III M) and 14% were in Social Classes IV and V. Among fifteen year olds the figures were similar, although there were a slightly lower proportion of children (38%) in Social Classes I, II and III N. Looking at the variation between countries, it can be seen that the main differences occur among the younger children. Among

Table 5.1 Social class of household

Social class of household	Age (years)			
	5	8	12	15
	%	%	%	%
England				
I, II, III N	44	42	37	39
III M	35	34	36	34
IV, V	14	17	17	17
Not given	7	7	10	10
All households	100	100	100	100
Wales				
I, II III N	37	34	37	37
III M	37	35	37	38
IV, V	20	23	22	19
Not given	6	8	4	6
All households	100	100	100	100
Scotland				
I, II, III N	34	33	31	35
III M	42	43	41	37
IV, V	16	18	19	20
Not given	8	6	9	8
All households	100	100	100	100
Northern Ireland				
I, II, III N	36	35	33	29
III M	39	33	38	34
IV, V	14	19	18	24
Not given	11	13	11	13
All households	100	100	100	100
United Kingdom				
I, II, III N	43	41	37	38
III M	36	35	36	35
IV, V	14	17	17	17
Not given	7	7	10	10
All households	100	100	100	100

For base numbers see Appendix A

the five and eight year olds, the highest proportion of children from Social Classes I, II and III N were found in England, the highest proportion from Social Class III M were from Scotland and the highest proportion from Social Classes IV and V were from Wales.

5.3 Active decay and household social class

The first measure of dental health that we look at in relation to household social class is that of active decay – that is, the current state of treatment need.

Table 5.2 shows the average number of decayed deciduous teeth. It can be seen that, in the United Kingdom, among the five and eight year olds, there was a lower average number of actively decayed teeth among Social Classes I, II and III N than among the

other social class groups. For example, on average among five year olds, twice as many teeth were actively decayed among those from Social Classes III manual, IV and V, than among Social Classes I, II and III N.

Children from England had the lowest average number of actively decayed deciduous teeth in all social class groups and it can be seen that, though in England those children from Social Classes IV and V were in the worst position, their average number of deciduous teeth with active decay was the same as the average number of deciduous teeth with active decay seen among the children from Social Classes I, II and III N in Wales.

Among the five year olds, children in each social class group in Scotland and Northern Ireland had a higher average number of actively decayed deciduous teeth than their counterparts in Wales. Among the eight year olds however, there was very little difference in this average between children in Wales, Scotland or Northern Ireland in Social Classes I, II and III N. There was, in fact, among the eight year olds very little difference in the average number of actively decayed teeth in each of the social class groups between children in Northern Ireland and children in Wales.

Looking at the average number of decayed permanent teeth among the older children in the United Kingdom, (Table 5.3) it can be seen that there was not much variation between the social class groups as was found in the average number of decayed deciduous teeth. It can also be seen that, in fact, there was very little

difference in the average number of actively decayed permanent teeth in each of the social class groups between children in England and in Wales.

It can be seen that those children with the worst averages in England and in Wales were still better off than the groups with the best averages in Scotland and Northern Ireland. In Northern Ireland, among the oldest children in Social Classes IV and V there were particularly high average number of permanent teeth with active decay.

5.4 Filled (otherwise sound) teeth and household social class

In this section, we look at the average number of filled (otherwise sound) teeth according to household social class. As we have said, in previous chapters, the decision to fill a decayed tooth may depend on whether or not the tooth is permanent or deciduous. To maintain a full dentition into adult life, decayed permanent teeth should be filled, if possible, rather than extracted. In the case of deciduous teeth, it is known that they will exfoliate naturally, and thus the decision may be taken not to fill the tooth.

Table 5.4 shows the average number of filled (otherwise sound) deciduous teeth by household social class. This average did not vary greatly between the different social class groups in the United Kingdom, although among the youngest children there was a slightly higher average number of filled deciduous teeth among those from Social Classes IV and V.

Table 5.2 Average number of decayed deciduous teeth by social class of household

Social class of household	Age (years)			
	5	8	12	15
England				
I, II, III N	0.6	0.8	0.1	–
III M	1.4	1.1	0.2	–
IV, V	1.6	1.4	0.2	–
All households	1.1	1.0	0.2	–
Wales				
I, II, III N	1.6	1.3	0.3	–
III M	1.9	1.6	0.4	–
IV, V	2.1	1.9	0.3	–
All households	1.8	1.5	0.3	–
Scotland				
I, II, III N	2.2	1.5	0.1	–
III M	2.9	2.1	0.3	–
IV, V	3.0	2.5	0.2	–
All households	2.6	2.0	0.2	–
Northern Ireland				
I, II, III N	2.5	1.4	0.2	–
III M	3.4	1.7	0.2	–
IV, V	*	2.1	0.4	–
All households	3.0	1.8	0.3	–
United Kingdom				
I, II, III N	0.8	0.9	0.1	–
III M	1.6	1.3	0.3	–
IV, V	1.8	1.5	0.2	–
All households	1.3	1.2	0.2	–

* *Average numbers not given for bases under 30*
  For base numbers see Appendix A

Table 5.3 Average number of actively decayed permanent teeth by social class of household

Social class of household	Age (years)			
	5	8	12	15
England				
I, II, III N	–	0.2	0.5	0.7
III M	–	0.3	0.5	0.9
IV, V	–	0.5	0.7	1.0
All households	–	0.3	0.6	0.9
Wales				
I, II, III N	–	0.2	0.5	0.9
III M	–	0.3	0.7	1.1
IV, V	–	0.3	0.7	1.3
All households	–	0.3	0.7	1.2
Scotland				
I, II, III N	–	0.5	0.7	1.3
III M	–	0.6	1.0	1.5
IV, V	–	0.8	1.5	1.8
All households	–	0.6	1.1	1.5
Northern Ireland				
I, II, III N	0.1	0.5	1.1	1.4
III M	–	0.7	1.4	2.3
IV, V	*	0.7	2.1	2.4
All households	0.1	0.7	1.5	2.1
United Kingdom				
I, II, III N	–	0.2	0.5	0.8
III M	–	0.3	0.6	1.0
IV, V	–	0.5	0.8	1.1
All households	–	0.3	0.6	1.0

* *Average numbers not given for bases under 30*
  For base numbers see Appendix A

Table 5.4 Average number of filled (otherwise sound) deciduous teeth by social class of household

Social class of household	Age (years)			
	5	8	12	15
England				
I, II, III N	0.4	1.1	0.3	–
III M	0.5	1.4	0.2	–
IV, V	0.8	1.0	0.2	–
All households	0.5	1.2	0.2	–
Wales				
I, II, III N	0.8	0.7	0.2	–
III M	0.6	1.2	0.2	–
IV, V	1.2	1.0	0.1	–
All households	0.8	1.3	0.2	–
Scotland				
I, II, III N	0.7	1.5	0.2	–
III M	0.6	1.1	0.2	–
IV, V	0.7	1.3	0.1	–
All households	0.6	1.3	0.2	–
Northern Ireland				
I, II, III N	1.0	1.5	0.2	–
III M	0.7	1.1	0.1	–
IV, V	*	0.9	0.2	–
All households	0.7	1.2	0.1	–
United Kingdom				
I, II, III N	0.5	1.2	0.2	–
III M	0.5	1.3	0.2	–
IV, V	0.9	1.0	0.2	–
All households	0.5	1.2	0.2	–

* Average numbers not given for bases under 30
For base numbers see Appendix A

Table 5.5 Average number of filled (otherwise sound) permanent teeth by household social class

Social class of household	Age (years)			
	5	8	12	15
England				
I, II, III N	–	0.4	1.9	3.9
III M	–	0.5	2.3	4.5
IV, V	–	0.4	2.0	4.4
All households	–	0.4	2.0	4.2
Wales				
I, II, III N	–	0.8	2.6	5.3
III M	–	0.6	2.1	4.7
IV, V	–	0.5	2.0	4.2
All households	–	0.6	2.3	4.8
Scotland				
I, II, III N	–	0.9	2.6	5.7
III M	–	0.8	3.1	6.2
IV, V	–	0.8	2.7	5.3
All households	–	0.8	2.9	5.8
Northern Ireland				
I, II, III N	–	1.1	3.0	6.7
III M	–	1.0	2.6	5.0
IV, V	*	0.8	2.2	6.3
All households	–	1.0	2.6	5.8
United Kingdom				
I, II, III N	–	0.5	2.0	4.2
III M	–	0.5	2.4	4.7
IV, V	–	0.5	2.1	4.5
All households	–	0.5	2.1	4.4

* Average numbers not given for bases under 30
For base numbers see Appendix A

Looking at the variation between the social class groups in the constituent countries of the United Kingdom, it can be seen that among the five year olds there was very little variation between the social classes in Scotland, while among children from England and children from Wales, those from Social Classes IV and V had the highest average number of filled deciduous teeth, and in Northern Ireland children from Social Classes I, II and III N had the highest average number of filled deciduous teeth.

In terms of the average number of filled permanent teeth (Table 5.5) there was little variation between children from different social class groups in the United Kingdom as a whole. In England and in Scotland the children with the highest average number of filled permanent teeth were from Social Class III M while in Wales and in Northern Ireland the highest averages were found among children from Social Classes I, II and III N.

5.5 Missing teeth and household social class
Permanent teeth which are missing because of decay represent the most serious type of decay experience as permanent teeth extracted will never be replaced.

In Table 5.6 we show how the average number of teeth extracted due to decay varied according to household social class. In the United Kingdom as a whole, the lowest average number of teeth missing due to decay was found among Social Classes I, II and III N and this was generally true in each of the separate countries. In each of the social class groups there was a lower average number of teeth missing due to decay in England than in the other countries but, in the case of Wales the differences were very small. Those children from Social Classes IV and V in Northern Ireland in this age group were again in the least favourable position. Compared with their counterparts in England, the average number of teeth missing due to decay was nearly three times higher (1.7 teeth compared with 0.6 teeth).

5.6 Known decay experience and household social class
Table 5.7 shows the average number of deciduous teeth that were either filled or decayed, for children in the different social class groups. In the United Kingdom as a whole, among the five year olds, those from Social Classes I, II and III N had the lowest average of decayed or filled deciduous teeth while those from Social Classes IV and V had the highest average. Among the eight year olds, those from Social Classes I, II and III N again had the lowest average number of decayed or filled deciduous teeth but there was no difference in this average between children from Social Class III manual and Social Classes IV and V.

The children from England from Social Classes I, II and III N had the lowest average number of decayed or filled deciduous teeth. Among five year olds from this group, for example, just one deciduous tooth on average was decayed or filled. Children from Social Classes IV and V in England were in at least as good a position, with regard to the average number of filled or

Table 5.6 Average number of permanent teeth missing due to decay by social class of household

Social class of household	Age (years)			
	5	8	12	15
England				
I, II, III N	–	–	0.2	0.4
III M	–	–	0.3	0.6
IV, V	–	0.1	0.3	0.6
All households	–	–	0.3	0.5
Wales				
I, II, III N	–	–	0.3	0.6
III M	–	–	0.2	0.8
IV, V	–	0.1	0.4	0.9
All households	–	–	0.3	0.8
Scotland				
I, II, III N	–	0.1	0.4	0.8
III M	–	–	0.5	1.2
IV, V	–	0.1	0.9	1.4
All households	–	0.1	0.6	1.1
Northern Ireland				
I, II, III N	–	–	0.6	0.9
III M	–	0.1	0.8	1.1
IV, V	*	0.2	0.8	1.7
All households	–	0.1	0.7	1.3
United Kingdom				
I, II, III N	–	–	0.2	0.4
III M	–	–	0.3	0.7
IV, V	–	0.1	0.4	0.7
All households	–	–	0.3	0.6

* Average numbers not given for bases under 30
For base numbers see Appendix A

Table 5.7 Average number of decayed or filled deciduous teeth by social class of household

Social class of household	Age (years)			
	5	8	12	15
England				
I, II, III N	1.0	1.9	0.4	–
III M	1.8	2.5	0.5	–
IV, V	2.4	2.4	0.4	–
All households	1.6	2.2	0.4	–
Wales				
I, II, III N	2.4	2.9	0.4	–
III M	2.4	2.8	0.6	–
IV, V	3.3	2.9	0.4	–
All households	2.6	2.8	0.5	–
Scotland				
I, II, III N	2.8	3.0	0.4	–
III M	3.4	3.3	0.4	–
IV, V	3.7	3.8	0.3	–
All households	3.2	3.3	0.4	–
Northern Ireland				
I, II, III N	3.5	2.9	0.3	–
III M	4.1	2.9	0.3	–
IV, V	*	3.0	0.5	–
All households	3.7	3.0	0.4	–
United Kingdom				
I, II, III N	1.3	2.1	0.4	–
III M	2.1	2.6	0.5	–
IV, V	2.6	2.6	0.4	–
All households	1.8	2.3	0.4	–

* Average numbers not given for bases under 30
For base numbers see Appendix A

decayed deciduous teeth, as children from Social Classes I, II and III N in the other countries. The five year olds from Northern Ireland from Social Classes I, II and III N were in a particularly poor position with an average of 3.5 deciduous teeth decayed or filled compared with an average of 2.8 among Social Classes I, II and III N in Scotland, 2.4 in Wales and 1.0 in England.

Table 5.8 shows the average number of permanent teeth with decay experience, that is, decayed, filled or missing due to decay, by household social class. In the United Kingdom, children from Social Classes I, II and III N had the lowest average decay experience, while there was no difference in the average decay experience of children from Social Class III manual and Social Classes IV and V. This was true of the children in England, while in Wales, children from Social Classes I, II and III N had the highest average decay experience.

In Scotland, the children with the highest average number of teeth with known decay experience were those from Social Classes III M, IV and V while in Northern Ireland, the children with the highest average number of teeth with known decay experience were those from Social Classes IV and V with the fifteen year olds being in a particularly poor position with an average of 10.4 permanent teeth with some known decay experience.

Table 5.8 Average number of decayed, filled or missing (due to decay) permanent teeth by social class of household

Social class of household	Age (years)			
	5	8	12	15
England				
I, II, III N	–	0.6	2.6	5.0
III M	–	0.7	3.1	6.0
IV, V	–	1.0	3.0	5.9
All households	–	0.7	2.9	5.6
Wales				
I, II, III N	–	1.0	3.3	6.8
III M	–	1.0	3.0	6.6
IV, V	–	0.9	3.1	6.4
All households	–	0.9	3.3	6.7
Scotland				
I, II, III N	–	1.4	3.7	7.8
III M	–	1.4	4.7	9.0
IV, V	–	1.7	5.2	8.5
All households	–	1.5	4.5	8.4
Northern Ireland				
I, II, III N	0.1	1.7	4.7	9.0
III M	–	1.8	4.8	8.4
IV, V	*	1.7	5.0	10.4
All households	0.1	1.9	4.8	9.2
United Kingdom				
I, II, III N	–	0.7	2.8	5.4
III M	–	0.9	3.3	6.3
IV, V	–	1.0	3.3	6.3
All households	–	0.8	3.1	5.9

* Average numbers not given for bases under 30
For base numbers see Appendix A

5.7 Dental attendance pattern

The previous section showed that the home background of a child in terms of his or her parents' social class is associated with that child's dental health in that, generally, those children from Social Classes I, II and III N were in the most fortunate position. Another factor which affects dental health is the regularity with which a child visits the dentist. We look in some detail at dental attendance patterns in Chapter 7 when we discuss the child's home environment but here we see how attendance patterns are related to the health of the teeth as measured by the survey examination.

Children who according to their parents had visited the dentist in the previous six months and whose last visit was for a check-up (whether or not they subsequently received treatment) were classified as regular dental attenders. Those who according to their parents had visited the dentist more than six months previously but whose visit had been for a check-up were classified as occasional attenders. Those whose last visit to the dentist had been because they had trouble with their teeth or because the school dentist had, after a school inspection, advised the parents that treatment was needed and those who had never visited a dentist were grouped together as those who attend only when having trouble with their teeth.

Table 5.9 shows the proportions of children with different dental attendance patterns in the countries of the United Kingdom. In the United Kingdom as a whole, in each of the four age groups, over half of the children were classified as regular attenders. For example, among eight year olds, 62% were regular attenders, 12% were occasional attenders and 26% attended only when having trouble with their teeth. These figures contained significant national variations. In each of the age groups, except the eight year olds, Northern Ireland had a considerably lower proportion of regular attenders and a higher proportion of children who visited the dentist only when having trouble with their teeth. For example, among fifteen year olds, 38% of children from Northern Ireland were classified as regular attenders compared with 61% in England, 58% in Wales and 52% in Scotland. In Northern Ireland, 41% of fifteen year olds attended the dentist only when having trouble with their teeth or had never attended the dentist compared with 20% of fifteen year olds in England, 23% in Wales and 31% in Scotland. Among five year olds and eight year olds the highest proportions classified as regular attenders and the lowest proportion of children who attended the dentist only when having trouble with their teeth were found in England. Scotland and Wales had similar proportions of children who, according to their parents, attended for a regular check-up but among the younger children Scotland had a higher proportion than Wales of children who attend the dentist only when having trouble with their teeth.

Table 5.9   Child's dental attendance pattern

Attendance pattern	Age (years)			
	5	8	12	15
	%	%	%	%
England				
Regular attenders	58	64	66	61
Occasional attenders	17	12	11	19
Only with trouble	25	24	23	20
All attenders	100	100	100	100
Wales				
Regular attenders	45	56	60	58
Occasional attenders	18	12	15	19
Only with trouble	37	32	25	23
All attenders	100	100	100	100
Scotland				
Regular attenders	43	53	60	52
Occasional attenders	11	9	12	17
Only with trouble	46	38	28	31
All attenders	100	100	100	100
Northern Ireland				
Regular attenders	26	51	41	38
Occasional attenders	18	15	20	21
Only with trouble	56	34	39	41
All attenders	100	100	100	100
United Kingdom				
Regular attenders	55	62	64	59
Occasional attenders	17	12	12	19
Only with trouble	28	26	24	22
All attenders	100	100	100	100

For base numbers see Appendix A

5.8 Active decay and attendance pattern

Table 5.10 shows the average number of actively decayed deciduous teeth among children according to dental attendance pattern. Among the five and eight year olds in the United Kingdom, those who were classified as regular attenders and those who were classified as occasional attenders had similar levels of actively decayed deciduous teeth while those who were said to attend only when having trouble with their teeth had a higher level. For example, among five year olds, there was an average of 0.9 actively decayed deciduous teeth among the regular attenders, 1.0 among the occasional attenders and 2.2 among those who attended the dentist only when having trouble with their teeth.

Among the five year olds, there were similar relationships in terms of the average number of decayed deciduous teeth between children with different attendance patterns in England and in Northern Ireland. In Scotland and Wales, however, those children who attended occasionally had a higher average number of actively decayed teeth than the regular attenders, but were still in a more favourable position than those who attended only when having trouble with their teeth.

Looking at the situation with regard to permanent teeth that were actively decayed (Table 5.11), it can be seen that, in each country, among the twelve and fifteen year olds, the regular attenders had a lower average number of actively decayed teeth than both the occasional attenders and those who attend only when having trouble with their teeth.

Table 5.10 Average number of actively decayed deciduous teeth by child's attendance pattern

Attendance pattern	Age (years)			
	5	8	12	15
England				
Regular attenders	0.8	0.8	0.2	–
Occasional attenders	0.8	0.9	0.2	–
Only with trouble	1.9	1.7	0.3	–
All attenders	1.1	1.0	0.2	–
Wales				
Regular attenders	1.1	1.1	0.3	–
Occasional attenders	2.0	*	0.2	–
Only with trouble	2.4	2.2	0.4	–
All attenders	1.8	1.5	0.3	–
Scotland				
Regular attenders	1.6	1.6	0.2	–
Occasional attenders	2.7	2.5	0.2	–
Only with trouble	3.6	2.4	0.3	–
All attenders	2.6	2.0	0.2	–
Northern Ireland				
Regular attenders	2.6	1.3	0.3	–
Occasional attenders	2.6	*	0.2	–
Only with trouble	3.4	2.2	0.2	–
All attenders	3.0	1.8	0.3	–
United Kingdom				
Regular attenders	0.9	0.9	0.2	–
Occasional attenders	1.0	1.1	0.2	–
Only with trouble	2.2	1.9	0.3	–
All attenders	1.3	1.2	0.2	–

* Means not given for bases under 30
For base numbers see Appendix A

Table 5.11 Average number of actively decayed permanent teeth by child's attendance pattern

Attendance pattern	Age (years)			
	5	8	12	15
England				
Regular attenders	–	0.2	0.4	0.6
Occasional attenders	–	0.3	0.8	0.9
Only with trouble	–	0.5	0.9	1.4
All attenders	–	0.3	0.6	0.9
Wales				
Regular attenders	–	0.2	0.4	0.7
Occasional attenders	–	*	0.7	1.2
Only with trouble	–	0.4	1.2	2.0
All attenders	–	0.3	0.7	1.2
Scotland				
Regular attenders	–	0.4	0.6	1.0
Occasional attenders	–	0.8	1.2	1.9
Only with trouble	–	0.8	1.9	2.2
All attenders	–	0.6	1.1	1.5
Northern Ireland				
Regular attenders	0.1	0.4	0.8	1.0
Occasional attenders	–	*	1.0	2.6
Only with trouble	0.1	1.0	2.4	2.7
All attenders	0.1	0.7	1.5	2.1
United Kingdom				
Regular attenders	–	0.2	0.4	0.6
Occasional attenders	–	0.3	0.8	1.0
Only with trouble	–	0.5	1.1	1.6
All attenders	–	0.3	0.6	1.0

* Means not given for bases under 30
For base numbers see Appendix A

Table 5.12 Average number of filled deciduous teeth by child's attendance pattern

Attendance pattern	Age (years)			
	5	8	12	15
England				
Regular attenders	0.6	1.3	0.3	–
Occasional attenders	0.2	0.8	0.2	–
Only with trouble	0.4	1.0	0.2	–
All attenders	0.5	1.2	0.2	–
Wales				
Regular attenders	1.1	1.4	0.2	–
Occasional attenders	0.1	*	0.1	–
Only with trouble	0.7	1.2	0.1	–
All attenders	0.8	1.3	0.2	–
Scotland				
Regular attenders	0.8	1.5	0.2	–
Occasional attenders	0.1	0.5	0.1	–
Only with trouble	0.6	1.1	0.1	–
All attenders	0.6	1.3	0.2	–
Northern Ireland				
Regular attenders	1.6	2.0	0.1	–
Occasional attenders	0.5	*	0.2	–
Only with trouble	0.5	0.6	0.1	–
All attenders	0.7	1.2	0.1	–
United Kingdom				
Regular attenders	0.7	1.3	0.3	–
Occasional attenders	0.2	0.8	0.2	–
Only with trouble	0.5	1.0	0.1	–
All attenders	0.5	1.2	0.2	–

* Means not given for bases under 30
For base numbers see Appendix A

Table 5.13 Average number of filled permanent teeth by child's attendance pattern

Attendance pattern	Age (years)			
	5	8	12	15
England				
Regular attenders	–	0.5	2.3	4.5
Occasional attenders	–	0.3	1.6	3.8
Only with trouble	–	0.5	1.8	3.9
All attenders	–	0.4	2.0	4.2
Wales				
Regular attenders	–	0.8	2.7	5.1
Occasional attenders	–	*	1.3	3.6
Only with trouble	–	0.5	1.9	4.8
All attenders	–	0.6	2.3	4.8
Scotland				
Regular attenders	–	1.0	2.9	6.6
Occasional attenders	–	0.6	2.4	4.8
Only with trouble	–	0.6	2.8	5.2
All attenders	–	0.8	2.9	5.8
Northern Ireland				
Regular attenders	–	1.4	3.7	7.0
Occasional attenders	–	*	2.5	4.4
Only with trouble	–	0.6	1.7	5.8
All attenders	–	1.0	2.6	5.8
United Kingdom				
Regular attenders	–	0.5	2.4	4.7
Occasional attenders	–	0.3	1.7	3.9
Only with trouble	–	0.5	1.9	4.1
All attenders	–	0.5	2.1	4.4

* Means not given for bases under 30
For base numbers see Appendix A

The average number of actively decayed teeth among those classified as regular attenders was similar in England and in Wales. In Scotland and Northern Ireland there were also similar levels of average actively decayed permanent teeth among the regular attenders.

Looking at the average number of actively decayed permanent teeth among those who were classified as visiting the dentist only when having trouble with their teeth, the lowest average was among these children in England followed, in order, by children from Wales, Scotland and Northern Ireland.

5.9 Filled (otherwise sound) teeth and attendance pattern

We have already noted that the decision to fill a decayed tooth may depend on whether the tooth is a deciduous tooth or a permanent tooth but the amount of fillings a child receives will depend on whether or not the child visits the dentist because, of course, dental decay cannot be treated except at the dental surgery.

Table 5.12 shows the average number of filled (otherwise sound) deciduous teeth. Not surprisingly, it can be seen that those children who were said to visit the dentist regularly, generally, have a higher average number of restored teeth. Those children who visit only occasionally have the lowest average number of restored teeth.

This was generally true in the case of filled permanent teeth (Table 5.13), although in England there was little difference between the average number of filled permanent teeth among those who were said to attend the dentist occasionally and those who were said to attend only when having trouble with their teeth, and among twelve year olds in Northern Ireland there was a higher average number of filled permanent teeth among the occasional attenders than among those who attend only when having trouble with their teeth.

5.10 Missing teeth and attendance pattern

Table 5.14 shows the average number of permanent teeth missing due to decay. As we have seen in previous chapters, there are higher numbers of teeth missing due to decay in Scotland and Northern Ireland, than in England and Wales but within the countries there were no very large differences between children of different attendance patterns (except among the fifteen year olds in Northern Ireland where the occasional attenders were in a comparatively fortunate position with an average number of missing teeth that was half that seen among the regular attenders and those who attend only when having trouble with their teeth).

5.11 Known decay experience and attendance pattern

Table 5.15 shows the average number of deciduous teeth that were decayed or filled. It can be seen that in all the countries but Northern Ireland, the highest average was seen among those children who were said to attend the dentist only when having trouble with their teeth or never. In Northern Ireland, however, it

Table 5.14 Average number of permanent teeth missing due to decay by child's attendance pattern

Attendance pattern	Age (years)			
	5	8	12	15
England				
Regular attenders	–	–	0.2	0.4
Occasional attenders	–	–	0.2	0.4
Only with trouble	–	0.1	0.4	0.8
All attenders	–	–	0.3	0.5
Wales				
Regular attenders	–	0.1	0.3	0.7
Occasional attenders	–	*	0.3	0.7
Only with trouble	–	–	0.5	0.9
All attenders	–	–	0.3	0.8
Scotland				
Regular attenders	–	–	0.5	1.1
Occasional attenders	–	0.1	0.3	1.3
Only with trouble	–	0.1	0.7	1.1
All attenders	–	0.1	0.6	1.1
Northern Ireland				
Regular attenders	–	–	0.6	1.4
Occasional attenders	–	*	0.8	0.7
Only with trouble	–	0.2	0.8	1.5
All attenders	–	0.1	0.7	1.3
United Kingdom				
Regular attenders	–	–	0.2	0.5
Occasional attenders	–	–	0.3	0.5
Only with trouble	–	0.1	0.4	0.8
All attenders	–	–	0.3	0.6

* Means not given for bases under 30
For base numbers see Appendix A

Table 5.15 Average number of decayed or filled deciduous teeth by child's attendance pattern

Attendance pattern	Age (years)			
	5	8	12	15
England				
Regular attenders	1.4	2.1	0.4	–
Occasional attenders	1.0	1.7	0.4	–
Only with trouble	2.4	2.8	0.5	–
All attenders	1.6	2.2	0.4	–
Wales				
Regular attenders	2.2	2.5	0.4	–
Occasional attenders	2.1	*	0.3	–
Only with trouble	3.1	3.3	0.5	–
All attenders	2.6	2.8	0.5	–
Scotland				
Regular attenders	2.4	3.1	0.4	–
Occasional attenders	2.8	3.1	0.3	–
Only with trouble	4.2	3.5	0.4	0.1
All attenders	3.2	3.3	0.4	–
Northern Ireland				
Regular attenders	4.3	3.2	0.4	–
Occasional attenders	3.1	*	0.3	–
Only with trouble	3.9	2.8	0.3	–
All attenders	3.7	3.0	0.4	–
United Kingdom				
Regular attenders	1.6	2.2	0.4	–
Occasional attenders	1.2	1.9	0.4	–
Only with trouble	2.7	2.9	0.5	–
All attenders	1.8	2.3	0.4	–

* Means not given for bases under 30
For base numbers see Appendix A

was the regular attenders who had the highest average number of decayed or filled deciduous teeth. Reference back to Tables 5.10 and 5.12 show that the reason for this relatively high average among the regular attenders in Northern Ireland was affected by the relatively high average number of filled deciduous teeth in this group.

Table 5.16 Average number of decayed, filled or missing (due to decay) permanent teeth by attendance pattern

Attendance pattern	Age (years)			
	5	8	12	15
England				
Regular attenders	–	0.6	2.8	5.5
Occasional attenders	–	0.6	2.6	5.0
Only with trouble	–	1.0	3.1	6.0
All attenders	–	0.7	2.9	5.6
Wales				
Regular attenders	–	1.0	3.4	6.5
Occasional attenders	–	*	2.3	5.5
Only with trouble	–	0.9	3.6	7.7
All attenders	–	0.9	3.3	6.7
Scotland				
Regular attenders	–	1.4	4.0	8.6
Occasional attenders	–	1.5	3.9	7.9
Only with trouble	–	1.6	5.4	8.5
All attenders	–	1.5	4.5	8.4
Northern Ireland				
Regular attenders	0.1	1.8	5.2	9.4
Occasional attenders	–	*	4.4	7.7
Only with trouble	0.1	1.9	4.9	10.0
All attenders	0.1	1.9	4.8	9.2
United Kingdom				
Regular attenders	–	0.7	3.0	5.8
Occasional attenders	–	0.7	2.8	5.3
Only with trouble	–	1.1	3.4	6.6
All attenders	–	0.8	3.1	5.9

* Means not given for bases under 30
For base numbers see Appendix A

From Table 5.16 it can be seen that, in the United Kingdom as a whole, children who were said to visit the dentist only when having trouble with their teeth had the highest average number of permanent teeth with known decay experience and, among the oldest children, the occasional attenders had the lowest average. This was true among the fifteen year olds in each of the constituent countries of the United Kingdom.

Among the twelve year olds in each of the constituent countries except Northern Ireland, those children who visited the dentist only when having trouble with their teeth had the highest average number of permanent teeth with known decay experience. In England and in Scotland, among the twelve year olds there was no difference in this average between those children who were said to be regular attenders and those who were said to be occasional attenders. In Northern Ireland, among the twelve year olds, there was a slightly higher average number of permanent teeth with known decay experience among the regular attenders than among the other children.

The table again emphasises the relatively poor position of the children in Scotland and Northern Ireland with regard to known decay experience.

5.12 Summary
In Wales, Scotland and Northern Ireland children from Social Classes I, II and III N had less evidence of decay experience than children from other social classes in the same country but they had more teeth involved with decay than was so among children of the same social class in England.

More than half of the children in the United Kingdom were said, by their parents to have visited a dentist for a check-up in the last six months. About a quarter were said to go to the dentist only when they had trouble with their teeth or not at all. Children in England were more likely than children elsewhere to attend regularly for a check-up.

The children who only go to the dentist when they have trouble with their teeth tended to have a higher number of actively decayed teeth than those who go for check-ups. Those who go for check-ups had more restored teeth than those who go only when they have some trouble. In terms of the decay experience for permanent teeth there was not much difference for the 15 year olds between the attendance groups. In all of the countries those who go for an occasional check-up had the lowest average number of teeth affected by disease. It is not possible to tell from survey results the extent to which attendance patterns have been selected on the basis of the children's pre-disposition to decay.

6 Dental background and dental decay, 1973 and 1983

6.1 Introduction

In the report on the 1973 survey, results were presented to establish the relationship between a child's dental health and the frequency with which they visited the dentist. In the previous chapter we saw how dental attendance patterns were related to dental health in the United Kingdom in 1983 and in this chapter we look at whether this relationship changed in England and Wales between 1973 and 1983.

As in 1973, in 1983 we defined attendance pattern in terms of how recently children had visited the dentist and the reason given by the parents for the last visit to the dentist. Regular attenders were defined as those whose last visit to the dentist, according to their parents, was for a check-up, whether or not they had subsequently received treatment, and was within the previous six months. Occasional attenders were those whose last visit had been for a check-up but had been longer ago than six months. Those children who had never been to the dentist, together with those whose parents had said that the child's last visit had been because they had had trouble with their teeth or because the school dentist had said that they should attend, were classed as children who attended the dentist only when having trouble with their teeth.

Before looking at how attendance pattern and dental health are related we look briefly at how the frequency of visiting the dentist changed between 1973 and 1983 (Table 6.1). The changes in attendance patterns and attitudes towards dentistry are discussed in more detail in Chapter 8.

The table shows that the proportion of children who attended the dentist for a regular check-up was larger in each of the age groups in 1983 than it had been in 1973. For example, among twelve year olds in 1973, 53% went to the dentist for a regular check-up, compared with 64% in 1983. In this chapter we look at changes in dental health within each of the attendance pattern groups.

6.2 Decay experience of the deciduous dentition

Table 6.2 shows the average number of actively decayed deciduous teeth per child in 1973 and 1983 according to dental attendance pattern. Among the five year olds in each of the attendance pattern groups, this average was lower in 1983 by at least one tooth with the largest difference being seen among the regular attenders where there was an average of 2.2 decayed deciduous teeth in 1973 compared with 0.8 in 1983. Even among the children who attended the dentist only when having trouble with their teeth or not at all the average number of actively decayed teeth among five year olds had decreased from 3.1 to 2.0.

Among eight year olds there was also a lower average number of actively decayed teeth in 1983 than in 1973, although in this age group, the decrease among the children who were said to visit the dentist only when having trouble with their teeth, was relatively small (2.2 teeth in 1973 compared with 1.8 teeth in 1983). Generally, in terms of the average number of deciduous teeth which were actively decayed, children who, in 1983, attended only when having trouble with their teeth were in a similar position to the regular attenders in 1973.

We saw in Chapter 4 that overall there has been very little change in the average number of filled (otherwise sound) deciduous teeth between 1973 and 1983. Table 6.3 shows that, within each of the individual attendance pattern groups there was little change in this figure between 1973 and 1983 except for a very small decrease in the average number of filled deciduous teeth among the regular attenders.

Table 6.1   Children's dental attendance patterns: England and Wales 1973 and 1983

Attendance pattern	Age (years)							
	5		8		12		14	15
	1973	1983	1973	1983	1973	1983	1973	1983
	%	%	%	%	%	%	%	%
Regular attenders	39	57	51	62	53	64	48	59
Occasional attenders	8	19	10	12	15	14	19	21
Only with trouble	53	24	39	24	32	22	33	20
All attenders	100	100	100	100	100	100	100	100

For base numbers see Appendix A

Table 6.2 Average number of actively decayed deciduous teeth by children's attendance pattern: England and Wales 1973 and 1983

Attendance pattern	Age (years)							
	5		8		12		14	15
	1973	1'83	1973	1983	1973	1983	1973	1983
Regular attenders	2.2	0.8	1.8	0.8	0.3	0.2	–	–
Occasional attenders	1.9	0.9	2.2	1.0	0.2	0.2	–	–
Only with trouble	3.1	2.0	2.2	1.8	0.4	0.3	–	–

For base numbers see Appendix A

Table 6.3 Average number of filled (otherwise sound) deciduous teeth by children's attendance pattern: England and Wales 1973 and 1983

Attendance pattern	Age (years)							
	5		8		12		14	15
	1973	1983	1973	1983	1973	1983	1973	1983
Regular attenders	1.1	0.7	1.6	1.3	0.2	0.3	–	–
Occasional attenders	0.2	0.2	0.9	0.8	0.1	0.2	–	–
Only with trouble	0.5	0.5	0.8	1.0	0.1	0.2	–	–

For base numbers see Appendix A

Table 6.4 Average number of decayed deciduous teeth and filled deciduous teeth by children's attendance pattern: England and Wales 1973 and 1983

Attendance pattern	Age (years)							
	5		8		12		14	15
	1973	1983	1973	1983	1973	1983	1973	1983
Regular attenders	3.3	1.5	3.4	2.1	0.5	0.4	–	–
Occasional attenders	2.1	1.1	3.1	1.8	0.3	0.4	–	–
Only with trouble	3.6	2.4	3.0	2.8	0.6	0.5	–	–

For base numbers see Appendix A

The average number of decayed deciduous teeth and filled deciduous teeth per child is shown in Table 6.4 for children with different attendance patterns. The table obviously reflects the changes that were noted in the previous tables, in particular that the largest improvements were noted among those with the best dental attendance patterns. Among five year olds, for example, the average number of deciduous teeth with known decay experience among the regular attenders had reduced by more than one half from 3.3 teeth in 1973 to 1.5 teeth in 1983.

6.3 Decay experience of the permanent dentition
The average number of permanent teeth with some active decay is shown in Table 6.5. The differences in these averages between 1973 and 1983 were substantial in each of the attendance pattern groups. Among the twelve year olds and among the oldest children this average had virtually halved in all of the groups. For example among twelve year old regular attenders there was an average of 1.0 actively decayed permanent teeth in 1973 compared with an average of 0.4 actively decayed teeth among the regular attenders in 1983. Among those twelve year olds who attend the dentist only when having trouble with their teeth the average was 2.3 in 1973 and 0.9 in 1983. The average number of actively decayed permanent teeth among those who, in 1983, attended the dentist only when having trouble with their teeth, was similar to the average number of actively decayed permanent teeth among regular attenders in 1973.

Table 6.6 shows the average number of filled (otherwise sound) permanent teeth among children with different attendance patterns. In 1973 it was shown that children who were said to visit the dentist for a regular check-up had a higher average number of filled permanent teeth than children who went to the dentist only when having trouble with their teeth. This was also the case in 1983, but in 1983 the disparity in the average number of filled teeth per child between the regular attenders and those who attend only when having trouble with their teeth had diminished. The average number of filled permanent teeth among regular attenders was considerably smaller in 1983 than in 1973, while the average number of filled teeth among those children who visited the dentist only when having trouble with their teeth remained virtually unchanged over the ten years. The reduction in the average number of filled teeth among the regular attenders is likely to reflect the reduction in dental disease over the ten year period. The fact that the average number of fillings among those who attend the dentist only when having trouble with their teeth has remained constant despite the reduction in disease is encouraging as it implies that a higher proportion of dental disease is being treated in 1983 than was the case in 1973.

Table 6.5 Average number of decayed permanent teeth by children's attendance pattern: England and Wales 1973 and 1983

Attendance pattern	Age (years)							
	5		8		12		14	15
	1973	1983	1973	1983	1973	1983	1973	1983
Regular attenders	–	–	0.6	0.2	1.0	0.4	1.3	0.6
Occasional attenders	–	–	0.7	0.3	1.5	0.8	1.9	0.9
Only with trouble	–	–	0.9	0.5	2.3	0.9	2.6	1.4

Table 6.6 Average number of filled (otherwise sound) permanent teeth by children's attendance pattern: England and Wales 1973 and 1983

Attendance pattern	Age (years)							
	5		8		12		14	15
	1973	1983	1973	1983	1973	1983	1973	1983
Regular attenders	–	–	1.3	0.5	3.6	2.3	6.1	4.5
Occasional attenders	–	–	0.8	0.3	2.2	1.5	4.1	3.8
Only with trouble	–	–	0.6	0.5	1.9	1.8	3.3	3.9

Table 6.7 Average number of permanent teeth missing due to decay by children's attendance pattern: England and Wales 1973 and 1983

Attendance pattern	Age (years)							
	5		8		12		14	15
	1973	1983	1973	1983	1973	1983	1973	1983
Regular attenders	–	–	0.1	–	0.5	0.2	0.7	0.4
Occasional attenders	–	–	–	–	0.7	0.2	0.7	0.4
Only with trouble	–	–	0.1	0.1	0.6	0.4	1.0	0.8

Table 6.8 Average number of permanent teeth with known decay experience by children's attendance pattern: England and Wales 1973 and 1983

Attendance pattern	Age (years)							
	5		8		12		14	15
	1973	1983	1973	1983	1973	1983	1973	1983
Regular attenders	–	–	2.0	0.7	5.1	2.9	8.1	5.6
Occasional attenders	–	–	1.5	0.6	4.4	2.6	6.7	5.1
Only with trouble	–	–	1.6	1.0	4.8	3.1	6.9	6.2

For base numbers for Tables 6.5 – 6.8 see Appendix A

Among the regular dental attenders and those who attend the dentist occasionally there was a decrease in the average number of permanent teeth missing due to decay (Table 6.7). For example, among twelve year olds in 1973 there was an average of 0.5 missing teeth among the regular attenders and 0.7 among the occasional attenders. The comparable figure in 1983 was 0.2 missing permanent teeth among both the regular and occasional attenders. There was no significant difference however between 1973 and 1983 in the average number of permanent teeth missing due to decay among the children who went to the dentist only when having trouble with their teeth.

Table 6.8 shows the variation in the known decay experience of the permanent dentition, that is, the average number of permanent teeth that were decayed, filled or missing due to decay. It can be seen that, although there were reductions in this average among children in each of the attendance pattern groups, the largest reductions were seen between the regular attenders in 1973 and in 1983. Among twelve year olds for example, the average number of teeth with known decay experience among the regular attenders was 2.9 teeth in 1983 compared with 5.1 teeth in 1973. Among the oldest children in 1973, the average number of permanent teeth with known decay experience was higher among the regular attenders than among those who attend the dentist only when having trouble with their teeth (due to the relatively high number of filled teeth among the regular attenders). However, in 1983, the situation of the oldest children was reversed and it was the children who attended only when having trouble with their teeth who had the highest average number of permanent teeth with known decay experience.

6.4 Summary

Over the last ten years there has been an increase in the number of children said to be going to the dentist for a regular check-up. The change was particularly marked among five year olds.

Active decay in deciduous teeth was at a much lower level in 1983 than 1973 and among the five year olds and 8 year olds those who go to the dentist for a regular check-up showed the greatest improvement. There was no significant difference between the average number of filled deciduous teeth among children in 1973 and in 1983.

The average number of actively decayed permanent teeth in 1983 was about half the level of 1973. The number of teeth involved was greater for those who were not in the habit of going to the dentist for a check-up but there were improvements for people in each attendance pattern. The average number of filled permanent teeth had gone down, over ten years, among those who go for dental check-ups, but was the same level or higher for those who only go once they have got trouble. The average number of permanent teeth extracted for decay reasons had gone down between 1973 and 1983 for all attendance patterns but the difference was greater for those who said they go for a dental check-up.

When the contributions made from active decay, filled teeth and those extracted because of decay are amalgamated to show the total decay experience of the permanent dentition it can be seen that although there were improvements in each attendance pattern the largest improvements over the ten years were among regular attenders.

7 Dental treatment and care

7.1 Introduction

In previous chapters, information relating to the current condition of the children's teeth as assessed by the dental examiner, was presented. Although the current state also gives an indication of past treatment, it does not give a complete picture of a child's dental history. In this chapter we look at the dental experiences of children in the United Kingdom in 1983 over their whole lives to date as reported by the parents on the postal questionnaires.

In addition we look at certain dental attitudes expressed by the parents and at the care that the children take of their teeth.

7.2 Treatment experience

Children's teeth may be affected by dental decay long before they start school so one would hope to find that by the age of five all the children in our sample had visited a dentist. Table 7.1 shows what proportion of the children in the four age groups had never visited a dentist. In the United Kingdom as a whole there were just 14% of five year olds who had never visited a dentist and this proportion decreased substantially between the ages of five and eight, while among fifteen year olds just 1% had never visited a dentist.

Table 7.1 Proportion of children who had never visited the dentist by social class of household

Social class of household	Age (Years)			
	5	8	12	15
England				
I, II, IIIN	10%	3%	1%	–
IIIM	15%	3%	3%	1%
IV, V	16%	10%	2%	1%
All households	13%	4%	2%	1%
Wales				
I, II, IIIN	8%	–	1%	–
IIIM	16%	8%	1%	1%
IV, V	19%	4%	2%	–
All households	16%	4%	1%	1%
Scotland				
I, II, IIIN	10%	2%	1%	1%
IIIM	17%	7%	1%	1%
IV, V	29%	1%	2%	2%
All households	17%	4%	1%	1%
Northern Ireland				
I, II, IIIN	23%	11%	3%	–
IIIM	25%	2%	6%	2%
IV, V	*	6%	5%	–
All households	29%	7%	5%	1%
United Kingdom				
I, II, IIN	10%	3%	1%	–
IIIM	15%	4%	3%	1%
IV, V	18%	9%	2%	1%
All households	14%	4%	2%	1%

* Percentages not given for bases of 30 or less
For base numbers see Appendix A

It can be seen from the table that the children from England had the lowest proportion who had never visited the dentist (13% among the five year olds), Wales and Scotland had similar percentages (16% and 17% respectively among the five year olds) and that the children from Northern Ireland had comparatively high proportions that had never visited the dentist (29% among the five year olds).

Among children from different social class groups, it was those from Social Classes I, II and IIIN who were most likely to have visited a dentist at some time in their lives. In England and in Wales, among the five year olds, those from Social Class IIIM and Social Classes IV and V were similar in terms of the proportion who had never visited the dentist. In Scotland however, on this issue, those from Social Class III M occupied an intermediate position and those from Social Classes IV and V were in a less favourable position (29% of five year olds from Social Classes IV and V had never visited a dentist). The number of five year olds in Northern Ireland from Social Classes IV and V was too small to permit separate analysis but it can be seen that, even among Social Classes I, II and IIIN in Northern Ireland, the proportion of children who had never visited a dentist was high.

A further indication of dental health which was collected from the parents was the type of treatment that the children had received at the dentist over the whole of his or her life so far. This will differ from the dental examiners assessment of current dental health in that it will include treatment carried out to teeth that were no longer in the mouth by the time of the examination.

Table 7.2 shows the proportion of children who had visited the dentist and who had not had any teeth filled or extracted at the dentists. Not surprisingly, this figure varied considerably between the age groups from 53% of five year olds to just 4% of fifteen year olds. Major variations in this proportion between groups of children with different background characteristics were confined to the five and eight year olds. Among five year olds in the United Kingdom, the highest proportion of children who had been to the dentist but not had any fillings or extractions was found among children from Social Classes I, II and IIIN (61%) and the lowest proportion among children from Social Classes IV and V (37%). Among eight year olds however, the proportion was still highest among Social Classes I, II and IIIN but children from Social Class III M and Social Classes IV and V had equal proportions.

As with previous indicators of dental health, the children from England were in the best position with 56% of five year olds who had visited the dentist having had neither a filling nor an extraction. Among five year olds, Northern Ireland was in the least favourable position with proportionately half as many children as in England who had attended the dentist without receiving a filling or having an extraction. Also among five year olds, there was very little difference overall between this proportion in Wales and in Scotland.

Table 7.2   Proportion of children who had visited the dentist and had never had an extraction or filling by social class of household

Social class of household	Age (years)			
	5	8	12	15
England				
I, II, IIIN	65%	32%	10%	6%
IIIM	52%	23%	7%	3%
IV, V	40%	24%	2%	5%
All households	56%	28%	8%	5%
Wales				
I, II, IIIN	38%	17%	12%	3%
IIIM	40%	20%	3%	2%
IV, V	25%	15%	4%	6%
All-households	35%	18%	7%	3%
Scotland				
I, II, IIIN	46%	13%	8%	1%
IIIM	31%	8%	2%	1%
IV, V	29%	10%	2%	3%
All households	37%	10%	5%	2%
Northern Ireland				
I, II, IIIN	39%	16%	7%	2%
IIIN	28%	12%	4%	2%
IV, V	*	9%	5%	4%
All households	27%	13%	5%	4%
United Kingdom				
I, II, IIIN	61%	29%	10%	5%
IIIM	49%	22%	6%	3%
IV, V	37%	22%	6%	5%
All households	53%	26%	7%	4%

* Percentages not given for bases of 30 or less
For base numbers see Appendix A

However, children from Social Classes I, II and IIIN in Scotland were in a better position than their counterparts in Wales, while the reverse was true among five year olds from Social Class IIIM.

As it has been shown that after the age of eight, only a small minority of children had not received treatment in the form of fillings or extractions, it is of interest to look at the variations in the type of treatment received.

Table 7.3 shows the proportions of children who, according to their parents, had ever had a tooth extracted. This proportion increased from 11% of the five year olds to 71% of the fifteen year olds in the United Kingdom. Again it was the children from England who were in the most favourable position. Among five year olds there were particularly noticeable differences in the proportion of children who had ever had a tooth extracted varying from 9% in England to 14% in Wales, 25% in Scotland and 27% in Northern Ireland.

Table 7.3   Proportion of children who have ever had extractions by social class of household

Social class of household	Age (years)			
	5	8	12	15
England				
I, II, IIIN	5%	37%	63%	64%
IIIM	10%	40%	63%	75%
IV, V	14%	45%	67%	73%
All households	9%	39%	64%	70%
Wales				
I, II, IIIN	15%	39%	68%	77%
IIIM	9%	49%	71%	76%
IV, V	22%	53%	80%	74%
All households	14%	47%	72%	75%
Scotland				
I, II, IIIN	22%	56%	71%	78%
IIIM	30%	63%	81%	83%
IV, V	22%	68%	81%	78%
All households	25%	63%	77%	80%
Northern Ireland				
I, II, IIIN	23%	48%	80%	89%
IIIM	30%	67%	83%	84%
IV, V	*	67%	75%	93%
All households	27%	60%	80%	87%
United Kingdom				
I, II, IIIN	7%	38%	64%	66%
IIIM	12%	43%	66%	76%
IV, V	15%	48%	69%	74%
All households	11%	42%	66%	71%

* Percentages not given for bases of 30 or less
For base numbers see Appendix A

Table 7.4   Proportion of children who have ever had a filling by social class of household

Social class of household	Age (years)			
	5	8	12	15
England				
I, II, IIIN	24%	55%	81%	91%
IIIM	27%	64%	82%	90%
IV, V	39%	49%	77%	88%
All Households	27%	57%	81%	90%
Wales				
I, II, IIIN	45%	73%	84%	92%
IIIM	37%	60%	86%	93%
IV, V	47%	66%	81%	82%
All households	41%	64%	84%	90%
Scotland				
I, II, IIIN	33%	76%	86%	95%
IIIM	36%	70%	90%	96%
IV, V	35%	74%	83%	88%
All households	33%	72%	86%	93%
Northern Ireland				
I, II, IIIN	31%	63%	77%	93%
IIIM	28%	71%	73%	84%
IV, V	*	58%	65%	87%
All households	29%	63%	72%	87%
United Kingdom				
I, II, IIIN	26%	57%	82%	92%
IIIM	29%	65%	83%	91%
IV, V	39%	53%	77%	87%
All households	29%	58%	81%	90%

* Percentages not given for bases of 30 or less
For base numbers see Appendix A

The proportions of children who had ever had a tooth filled was higher than those who had ever had an extraction (Table 7.4). By the time the age of fifteen had been reached, nine out of ten of the children had, at some time in their lives, had a filling. Among the five and eight year olds the children from England had the lowest proportion who had ever had a filling while among the older children the lowest proportions were seen in Northern Ireland. Among five year olds there was a comparatively high proportion of children from Wales who had ever had a filling (41%) compared with the other countries (27% in England, 33% in Scotland and 29% in Northern Ireland), but this national variation was not apparent in the other age groups.

In terms of social class, there was little clear variation between the proportions of children in the different groups who had ever had a filling.

It will be noted from Table 7.4 that the proportions of parents of five year olds who said that their child had ever had a filling was slightly higher than the proportions of five year olds with a filled tooth shown in Chapter 3. However the filled teeth shown in that chapter were teeth that were filled and otherwise sound. The teeth that had unsound fillings or had other areas of decay were classified as actively decayed. We found that in general, parents of five year olds were, perhaps not suprisingly, accurate in their reporting of whether or not their child had had a filling. We could not make comparisons between the parent's answers and the dental data for the older children for some of the teeth that the parent's said had been filled, may have exfoliated by the time of the examination.

7.3 Preferences for treatment
If children are to have a good chance of retaining their natural teeth for life, then it would be hoped that they would not have any of their permanent teeth extracted because of decay during childhood. We asked parents whether, if their child had a 'bad' permanent tooth, they would prefer it to be filled or extracted, and we asked this question separately about bad back teeth and bad front teeth. It is encouraging to see, in Table 7.5, that a high proportion of parents preferred their child to have a decayed permanent tooth filled rather than

extracted. This figure was higher in the case of front teeth than back teeth, indicating that some parents place importance on their child's appearance rather than hold an attidue that the loss of permanent teeth is an undesirable occurrence *per se*.

No national variation was seen in these figures but as can be seen from the table there was a variation according to the parent's social class with those from Social Classes IV and V being less likely to prefer a decayed tooth to be filled.

7.4 Dental care
We have seen that generally, the majority of parents are in favour of their children preserving their natural teeth rather than having them extracted if they cause pain. We were interested to know how parents thought they could help to preserve their children's teeth and asked the questions *'What do you think makes teeth decay (or go bad)?'* and *'What do you think can be done to stop teeth decaying (or going bad)?'*. It can be seen from Table 7.6 that all but 1% of the parents had a view on what caused dental decay and that the causes mentioned by the majority of parents were eating sweet things and not cleaning the teeth properly. A higher proportion of parents of five year olds than of fifteen year olds (78% compared with 68%) said that they thought that sweet things caused decay, but there was very little other variation with age in the answers given about the causes of decay. Apart from the two major reasons mentioned by the parents as the cause of decay, a wide variety of other reasons were given. A poor diet was mentioned by one in five of the parents as a cause of decay but none of the other reasons advanced were mentioned by more than one in ten of the parents.

Table 7.6   Parents suggested causes of tooth decay

'What do you think makes teeth decay (or go bad)?'	Age (years)			
	5	8	12	15
Sweet things	78%	75%	73%	68%
Not cleaning teeth properly	72%	69%	69%	73%
Poor diet	19%	19%	20%	19%
Hereditary	7%	8%	6%	6%
Not going to dentist	5%	5%	7%	6%
Lack of fluoride	1%	1%	1%	1%
Other specified answer	6%	7%	6%	6%
Don't know	1%	1%	1%	1% .

For bases see Appendix A

Table 7.5   Preferences for treatment of decayed permanent teeth by social class of household

Social class of household	Age (years)			
	5	8	12	15
Permanent back tooth	*Proportion of parents who would prefer the tooth to be filled*			
I, II, IIIN	95%	92%	93%	92%
IIIM	85%	87%	85%	84%
IV, V	78%	81%	76%	81%
All households	88%	87%	86%	87%
Permanent front tooth				
I, II, IIIN	94%	94%	97%	96%
IIIM	93%	92%	92%	95%
IV, V	88%	88%	85%	88%
All households	92%	92%	92%	93%

For base numbers see Appendix A

Table 7.7   Parents suggestions for preventing decay

'What do you think can be done to stop teeth decaying (or going bad)?'	Age (years)			
	5	8	12	15
Avoid sweet things	48%	42%	37%	37%
Clean teeth regularly	74%	75%	71%	74%
Have a balanced diet	28%	26%	27%	24%
Visit dentist regularly	31%	29%	30%	34%
More dental education	9%	8%	6%	6%
Preventive treatment at dentists	4%	4%	4%	3%
Use fluoride toothpaste/ tablets	8%	6%	5%	5%
Add fluoride to water	3%	1%	2%	2%
Fluoride (nothing else specified)	3%	3%	3%	3%
Other answers	5%	5%	4%	4%
Don't know	2%	2%	3%	2%

For bases see Appendix A

Table 7.7 shows the answers given by the parents when asked what they thought could be done to prevent teeth decaying. Because these questions were asked via a postal questionnaire rather than in a face-to-face interview, we were unable to know exactly what some of the answers given implied. For example, some parents wrote the answer 'fluoride' but did not say in what form they thought fluoride should be administered, while other parents were more specific and the different methods mentioned of administering fluoride are shown separately in the table. No parent, in fact mentioned more than one method of administering fluoride and thus the codes concerning fluoride shown in the table are additive: so, 14% of the parents of five year olds mentioned fluoride and 10% of the parents of eight year olds, twelve year olds and fifteen year olds mentioned fluoride in replying to this question.

About three quarters of parents said that they thought that cleaning the teeth regularly stopped teeth decaying, and this was by far the most common answer given. It is interesting to see that, though a very high proportion of parents said that they thought sweet things caused tooth decay, a much smaller proportion said that avoiding sweet things would prevent decay. (The proportion saying this declined from 48% among parents of five year olds to 37% among parents of fifteen year olds.) It would seem that though parents felt that eating sweet things caused decay, regular tooth brushing was able to counteract these harmful effects. About a quarter of the parents said that eating a balanced diet would prevent decay and around a third said that visiting the dentist regularly would prevent decay. It is, perhaps, surprising that such a relatively small proportion of parents specifically mentioned fluoride toothpaste as a method of preventing decay since there has, in recent years, been a large amount of television advertising promoting the use of fluoride in toothpaste as a preventive measure. It may have been, however, that those parents who answered that brushing the teeth prevented decay actually meant that brushing the teeth with a fluoride toothpaste prevented decay.

In the 1973 survey the parents of the children were asked the same two questions. The results are not strictly comparable as, in 1973, the questions were asked in a face-to-face interview rather than by post. However, it is of interest to see that, in 1973, as in 1983, a high proportion of parents said that sweet things caused decay but a considerably lower proportion said that lack of care of the teeth caused decay. The higher response in 1983 of answers mentioning not cleaning the teeth properly as a reason is likely to have been due to the increased emphasis in the media on the importance of tooth brushing.

As it has been shown that parents thought brushing the teeth was important in preventing tooth decay, it is interesting to see how often parents said their children brushed their teeth (or had them brushed for them).

In the United Kingdom, about one half of the parents said that their children brushed their teeth twice a day (Table 7.8). (This figure may not reflect the truth in that parents may be giving an acceptable answer rather than reporting the actual situation.) A slightly higher proportion of the fifteen year olds were reported as cleaning their teeth three or more times a day (12% compared with 4% in the other three age groups).

Table 7.8 Frequency of brushing the teeth

Frequency	Age (years)			
	5	8	12	15
England	%	%	%	%
Three or more times a day	3	4	5	12
Twice a day	67	62	62	61
Once a day	26	27	25	21
Less than once a day	3	5	6	4
Never	–	1	1	1
Don't know	–	1	1	1
All children	100	100	100	100
Wales				
Three or more times a day	3	2	6	13
Twice a day	58	64	56	57
Once a day	33	26	28	25
Less than once a day	6	7	7	5
Never	–	–	2	1
Don't know	1	1	1	–
All children	100	100	100	100
Scotland				
Three or more times a day	10	8	9	15
Twice a day	59	58	54	54
Once a day	25	26	25	23
Less than once a day	5	6	8	5
Never	1	1	2	2
Don't know	–	1	1	1
All children	100	100	100	100
Northern Ireland				
Three or more times a day	2	3	1	12
Twice a day	51	50	54	59
Once a day	36	38	34	19
Less than once a day	8	6	9	7
Never	1	2	1	1
Don't know	1	2	–	2
All children	100	100	100	100
United Kingdom				
Three or more times a day	4	4	4	12
Twice a day	53	52	51	46
Once a day	35	33	34	30
Less than once a day	7	7	10	8
Never	1	3	1	3
Don't know	–	1	1	1
All children	100	100	100	100

For bases see Appendix A

Looking at the variation between the countries of the United Kingdom, in the age groups five, eight and twelve, a significantly higher proportion of children in Northern Ireland were reported as brushing their teeth less than twice a day or never, compared with the other countries. For example, among eight year olds, 46% of children in Northern Ireland were said to brush their teeth less than twice a day or never, compared with 33% in each of the other countries. There was very

little difference, however, between the countries in the reported tooth brushing habits of the fifteen year olds.

Table 7.9 shows how the frequency of brushing the teeth is related to a child's dental health. It shows that the proportions of children in each age group recorded as having some active decay or some debris was lower among children who were said to brush their teeth twice a day or more often than among those who were said to brush their teeth less often than this.

However, one must be wary about making a direct link between more frequent brushing and better dental health. It is likely that children who are reported as brushing their teeth twice or more times a day come from a more dentally aware background than those who are said to brush their teeth once a day or less often. It is unlikely that solely tooth brushing habits caused the variation noted in the table.

Table 7.10 shows that, not surprisingly, virtually all the older children brush their own teeth while among the five year olds 43% had their teeth brushed with the aid of the parents. The most popular times for cleaning teeth were before going to school in the morning and before bed at night. Among the older children, as compared with the younger, a higher proportion cleaned their teeth before breakfast and a lower proportion cleaned them afterwards. For example, among fifteen year olds 25% brushed their teeth before breakfast and 65% after breakfast, compared with 12% and 72% respectively among the five year olds.

Finally in this section on dental care we look at whether or not any professional advice had been received about children's dental health. Table 7.11 shows the proportions of parents and/or children who had received some professional advice about the care of the children's teeth. The proportion who had received such advice increased from 48% in the case of five year olds to 61% for fifteen year olds. In each of the age groups a lower proportion of children from Northern Ireland had received dental advice than children from each of the other countries.

Table 7.9 Brushing the teeth and dental health

Reported frequency of brushing the teeth	Age (years)							
	5		8		12		15	
	Proportion of children with some current active decay							
Three or more times a day	*	27	45%	40	37%	61	36%	131
Twice a day	38%	490	48%	561	35%	673	39%	650
Once a day	46%	202	64%	249	47%	282	47%	236
Less than once a day	54%	32	70%	57	45%	85	58%	63
	Proportion of children with some debris							
Three or more times a day	*	27	49%	40	39%	61	33%	131
Twice a day	28%	490	50%	561	40%	673	44%	650
Once a day	28%	202	63%	249	62%	282	54%	236
Less than once a day	52%	32	72%	57	69%	85	70%	63

* *Percentages not given for bases of 30 or less*

Table 7.10 Who brushes children's teeth and when the teeth are brushed

	Age (years			
	5	8	12	15
Who brushes the teeth	%	%	%	%
Child	54	86	97	98
Parent with child	43	10	1	–
Other	1	1	–	–
Don't know	2	2	1	1
Never brushes teeth	–	1	1	1
All children	100	100	100	100
When teeth are brushed?				
Before breakfast	12%	15%	22%	25%
After breakfast	72%	70%	64%	65%
Midday	2%	2%	2%	5%
Before evening meal	1%	1%	–	1%
After evening meal	5%	4%	6%	13%
Before bed	81%	79%	77%	75%
At other times	2%	3%	3%	4%
Base	756	914	1,109	1,089

Table 7.11 Proportion who had received advice on child's dental care

	Age (years)			
	5	8	12	15
England	49%	58%	62%	61%
Wales	45%	57%	62%	56%
Scotland	48%	60%	66%	63%
Northern Ireland	33%	44%	53%	52%
United Kingdom	48%	57%	62%	61%

For bases see Appendix A

Table 7.12 Who received the dental advice

Who had received the advice	Age (years)			
	5	8	12	15
	%	%	%	%
Parent	21	19	16	14
Child	6	12	17	18
Parent and child	21	27	28	28
Never received advice	50	41	36	37
Don't know if advised	2	2	2	2
All parents	100	100	100	100

For bases see Appendix A

Table 7.13 Who gave the dental advice (for those who had received advice)

Who gave the dental advice	Age (years)			
	5	8	12	15
Dentist	83%	84%	82%	87%
Dental hygenist	15%	14%	16%	11%
Dental nurse	6%	7%	8%	7%
Health visitor	6%	2%	3%	3%
Teacher	6%	4%	3%	2%
Doctor	2%	2%	2%	2%
Other	4%	7%	6%	7%
Base	317	539	709	685

The proportion of parents who said that either the child alone or both the child and the parent had received dental advice increased with the age of the child, (Table 7.12), while the proportions who said that they alone had received advice about their child's dental health decreased with the age of the child.

Of those parents or children who said that they had received dental advice, over 80% had received this advice from the dentist (Table 7.13), while just over 10% had received the advice from the dental hygenist.

7.5 Visiting the dentist

In addition to the care that children take of their teeth at home, another aspect of dental health is the regularity or otherwise with which they visit the dentist. It has already been shown in Chapter 5 that children's dental attendance patterns are closely related to their dental health, as measured on the survey dental examination and in this section we present information concerning the frequency with which children visit the dentist and the types of dental service they have used.

As explained in Chapter 5 attendance patterns were derived by combining the parental responses to a question on length of time since previous dental visit and a question on the reason for that last visit. Regular dental attenders were defined as those whose last visit to the dentist had been for a check-up (whether or not they subsequently received any treatment) and was said to be within the previous six months. Occasional attenders were those whose last visit was longer ago than six months but was also for a check-up. Children who attended only when having trouble with their teeth were those whose last visit had been either because they had trouble with their teeth or because they had brought home a note after a school dental inspection that notified the parents that the child should attend a dentist. Also included in this latter category were those children who had never visited the dentist.

In the United Kingdom as a whole, attendance patterns varied little between the age groups. In each group the majority of children were regular dental attenders and about one quarter attended only when having trouble with their teeth (Table 7.14). There was however considerable national variation. There was a higher proportion of regular attenders in England than in any of the other countries, although among the fifteen year olds the difference between those from England and those from Wales was minimal. In terms of the proportion of regular attenders, children aged five, eight and twelve in Wales were similar to those in Scotland. Among all but the eight year olds, the children from Northern Ireland were much less likely to be regular attenders than children in the other countries. Among twelve year olds, for example, 40% of Northern Ireland children were regular attenders compared with 66% in England and 60% in both Wales and Scotland.

The dental habits and attitudes of the other people in a child's family have an influence on the child's dental care, in that those children who come from a dentally aware family are likely to demonstrate good dental habits. As, in the majority of cases, the mother has the main responsibility for looking after the child, we look, in Table 7.15 at how the mother's dental attendance pattern is related to the child's attendance pattern. The dental attendance pattern of the mothers was ascertained by asking the question, *'In general, do you go to the dentist for a regular check-up, an occasional check-up or only when you are having trouble with your teeth?'*.

Table 7.14 Children's dental attendance pattern

Attendance pattern	Age (years)			
	5	8	12	15
England	%	%	%	%
Regular attenders	58	64	66	61
Occasional attenders	17	12	11	19
Only with trouble	25	24	23	20
All attenders	100	100	100	100
Wales				
Regular attenders	45	56	60	58
Occasional attenders	18	12	15	19
Only with trouble	37	32	25	23
All attenders	100	100	100	100
Scotland				
Regular attenders	43	53	60	52
Occasional attenders	11	9	12	17
Only with trouble	46	38	28	31
All attenders	100	100	100	100
Northern Ireland				
Regular attenders	26	51	40	38
Occasional attenders	18	15	20	21
Only with trouble	56	34	39	41
All attenders	100	100	100	100
United Kingdom				
Regular attenders	55	62	64	59
Occasional attenders	17	12	12	19
Only with trouble	28	26	24	22
All attenders	100	100	100	100

For bases see Appendix A

Because the concept of attendance pattern is not relevant to those people who have lost all their natural teeth, the edentulous mothers are separated from the dentate in the table.

A very high proportion of children whose mothers were regular attenders were themselves regular attenders. For example among twelve year olds, 82% of children whose mothers were regular attenders were themselves regular attenders while among twelve year old children whose mother attended the dentist only when having trouble with their teeth, just 40% were regular attenders.

Similarly, the mothers of children who were said to attend only when having trouble with their teeth were more likely themselves to attend only when having trouble with their teeth.

Table 7.16 shows the age according to their parents that the children first attended a dentist. It can be seen that a much higher proportion of five year olds had visited the dentist before the age of five compared with the fifteen year olds. This variation is likely to be affected, in part, by the fact that the parents of the younger children were remembering a much more recent occurrence. However, we will see in the following chapter that, in England and Wales, there has been a change over the last ten years towards taking children to the dentist at an earlier age.

Table 7.15 Child's attendance pattern, by mother's attendance pattern

Mother's attendance pattern	Age (years)			
	5	8	12	15
	Proportion of children who are regular attenders			
Regular attenders	72% 434	77% 515	82% 546	75% 498
Occasional attenders	32% 141	44% 162	45% 190	44% 178
Only with trouble	26% 131	36% 154	40% 205	36% 205
Edentulous	* 20	43% 51	48% 38	53% 45
	Proportion of children who attend only when they have trouble with teeth			
Regular attenders	13% 434	13% 515	10% 546	9% 498
Occasional attenders	33% 141	36% 162	31% 190	25% 178
Only with trouble	59% 131	51% 154	41% 205	37% 208
Edentulous	* 20	40% 51	39% 38	29% 405

* Percentages not given for bases of 30 or less.

Table 7.16 Age first visited the dentist

Age at first visit (years)	Current age (years)			
	5	8	12	15
England	%	%	%	%
Less than 2	7	6	5	3
2, less than 3	19	19	13	12
3, less than 4	35	24	21	22
4, less than 5	19	17	18	17
5 or more	6	27	37	40
Never been	13	4	2	1
Don't know	2	3	4	6
All children	100	100	100	100
Wales				
Less than 2	5	2	5	3
2, less than 3	23	13	12	10
3, less than 4	27	23	20	15
4, less than 5	18	28	19	20
5 or more	10	25	40	44
Never been	16	4	1	1
Don't know	2	3	4	7
All children	100	100	100	100
Scotland				
Less than 2	7	5	4	4
2, less than 3	18	12	11	11
3, less than 4	28	30	24	17
4, less than 5	19	19	20	19
5 or more	11	28	37	44
Never been	17	4	1	1
Don't know	1	3	4	3
All children	100	100	100	100
Northern Ireland				
Less than 2	2	3	–	2
2, less than 3	11	8	3	2
3, less than 4	18	13	12	8
4, less than 5	25	18	14	15
5 or more	13	49	59	68
Never been	29	7	5	1
Don't know	1	4	8	5
All children	100	100	100	100
United Kingdom				
Less than 2	7	6	5	3
2, less than 3	19	18	13	11
3, less than 4	33	24	21	21
4, less than 5	19	18	18	18
5 or more	6	27	37	40
Never been	14	4	2	1
Don't know	1	3	4	6
All children	100	100	100	100

For bases see Appendix A

In the case of five year olds where the results are likely to be the most accurate, it can be seen that in terms of the proportion who attended the dentist aged less than four, England was in the best position (61%), Wales and Scotland were in similar positions (55% and 53% respectively) and Northern Ireland were in the worst position with just 31% of five year olds having visited the dentist at the age of three or earlier.

There was considerable variation in the proportion of children who had visited the dentist aged three or younger between children with differing backgrounds (Table 7.17). A much higher proportion of children whose mothers were regular attenders than of those whose mothers attended only when having trouble with their teeth, had visited the dentist when they were aged less than four. For example, among five year olds, 75% of children whose mothers were regular attenders had been to the dentist before the age of four compared with just 27% of children whose mothers visited the dentist only when having trouble with their teeth. Similarly, a higher proportion of children from Social Classes I, II and IIIN had been to the dentist before the age of four compared with children from Social Classes IV and V.

The majority of treatment received by children is provided either by the General Dental Service or the Community Dental Service, but some treatment may be supplied privately. Table 7.18 shows the variations in the types of service used by the children. In the United Kingdom as a whole, a third of the five year olds had received treatment from the General Dental Service only, 7% had received treatment from the Community Dental Service only, 4% had received treatment both from a General Dental Service dentist and the Community Dental Service, 1% had received some form of private treatment and 56% had not received any dental treatment. The take-up of each type of dental service increased among the older children and among fifteen year olds 57% had received treatment only from a General Dental Service dentist, 13% had received treatment solely from the Community Dental Service, 19% had used both types of services, 7% had received some private treatment and 3% had not received any dental treatment.

Table 7.17 Proportion of children who went to the dentist at age 3 or earlier by mother's dental attendance pattern and social class of household

	Children who went to the dentist at age 3 or earlier currently aged:			
	5	8	12	15
Mother's dental attendance pattern				
Regular attenders	75% 434	62% 515	54% 546	51% 498
Occasional attenders	45% 141	37% 162	25% 190	29% 178
Only with trouble	27% 131	18% 154	20% 205	17% 205
Edentulous	* 20	39% 51	24% 38	28% 45
Social class of household				
I, II, III Non manual	72% 321	63% 373	49% 407	47% 416
III Manual	55% 268	45% 315	35% 404	33% 378
IV, V	42% 108	25% 159	28% 191	23% 189

* Percentages not given for bases of 30 or less

Table 7.18 The type of service used

Services with which child has received treatment	Age (years)			
	5	8	12	15
England	%	%	%	%
General Dental Service only	31	44	55	57
Community Dental Service only	5	14	16	13
Community Dental Service and General Dental Service	3	10	16	18
Private treatment only	–	1	–	–
Private treatment and General Dental Service and/or Community Dental Service	1	6	7	8
Child not received treatment	59	25	6	4
All services	100	100	100	100
Wales				
General Dental Service only	39	44	57	54
Community Dental Service only	20	25	14	16
Community Dental Service and General Dental Service	6	11	17	22
Private treatment only	–	–	–	–
Private treatment and General Dental Service and/or Community Dental Service	1	7	5	4
Child not received treatment	34	13	7	3
All services	100	100	100	100
Scotland				
General Dental Service only	41	43	55	58
Community Dental Service only	13	16	14	13
Community Dental Service and General Dental Service	6	26	25	25
Private treatment only	–	–	–	–
Private treatment and General Dental Service and/or Community Dental Service	1	6	4	2
Child not received treatment	39	9	2	2
All services	100	100	100	100
Northern Ireland				
General Dental Service only	35	50	53	62
Community Dental Service only	10	16	14	7
Community Dental Service and General Dental Service	5	14	19	20
Private treatment only	–	–	1	–
Private treatment and General Dental Service and/or Community Dental Service	1	3	3	9
Child not received treatment	49	17	10	3
All services	100	100	100	100
United Kingdom				
General Dental Service only	32	44	55	57
Community Dental Service	7	15	16	13
Community Dental Service and General Dental Service	4	12	17	19
Private treatment only	–	–	–	–
Private treatment and General Dental Service and/or Community Dental Service	1	6	6	7
Child not received treatment	56	23	6	3
All services	100	100	100	100

For bases see Appendix A

Table 7.19 Type of treatment received privately

Type of treatment received privately	Age (years)			
	5	8	12	15
Preventive treatment	*	88%	70%	66%
Fillings	*	5%	10%	13%
Extractions	*	4%	10%	5%
Other treatment	*	4%	12%	19%
Base (those who had had private treatment)	11	56	70	78

* Percentages not given for bases of 30 or less

Among the younger children, the use of the Community Dental Service was relatively low in England. For example among five year olds, 8% had used this service either solely or in addition to a General Dental Service dentist compared with 26% in Wales, 19% in Scotland and 15% in Northern Ireland. Among the five and eight year olds, the use solely of the Community Dental Service for treatment was particularly high in Wales.

7.6 Private treatment
It was seen from Table 7.18 that a relatively small proportion of children had received private treatment but it is of interest to see the types of treatment that were being provided privately. Previous surveys of adult dental health[1,2] have shown that the majority of adults who chose to receive their treatment privately, received treatment that was readily available under the General Dental Service and it was therefore for reasons other than the types of treatment that were provided that made people choose to attend privately. However, this is not true for children. Table 7.19 shows that the vast majority of treatment provided privately was of the type that would not normally be available through the General Dental Service. Among eight year olds, for example, 88% of the treatment that had been provided privately was preventive treatment such as the application of fissure sealants. This compared with a level of just 5% for fillings, 4% for extractions and 4% for other types of treatment, which mainly comprised orthodontic work.

7.7 Summary

In the United Kingdom 14% of five year olds had never been to the dentist. It was much more common in Northern Ireland for children of this age not to have established the habit of going to the dentist. Encouraging youngsters to get used to going to the dentist was more common among children from Social Classes I, II and III N than among other social classes.

Over half of five year olds in the United Kingdom had visited a dentist but had had neither fillings nor extractions. This was so for 61% of five year olds in Social Classes I, II and III non-manual. Among the eight year olds a quarter had been to the dentist but never had any extractions or fillings done. By the age of twelve only 7% of children had been to the dentist without having any extractions or fillings.

Parents were asked whether, if their child had a bad back permanent tooth, they would prefer it to be filled or extracted; more than four out of five said they would prefer it to be filled.

When asked about what causes decay three quarters of the parents thought eating sweets causes decay and nearly as many said not cleaning the teeth properly causes decay. When asked what could be done to stop teeth from decaying, three quarters of the parents said cleaning teeth regularly but only about two out of five said that sweet things should be avoided.

About half of the children were said, by their parents, to brush their teeth twice a day. Children who were said not to brush their teeth as often as twice a day were more likely to have current active decay, and were more likely to have been recorded in the examination as having some debris on their teeth. It is possible that these associations were influenced by whether or not parents had a dentally aware attitude and were generally guiding and influencing their child's dental habits, than that the frequency of toothbrushing was alone responsible for the association. Attitudes towards dentistry were clearly important, for among children whose mothers were regular dental attenders, three quarters of the children were also regular attenders, whereas among those whose mothers only go to the dentist when they have trouble only about a third of the children were regular attenders.

References

[1] P Gray et al. *Adult dental health in England and Wales in 1968.* HMSO (1970).
[2] J E Todd, A M Walker and P Dodd. *Adult dental health, Volume 2: United Kingdom 1978.* HMSO (1982).

8 Dental treatment and care 1973 and 1983

8.1 Introduction
We have already seen a welcome reduction in tooth decay among children in 1983 and in this chapter we see that this improvement is associated with better dental habits in terms of cleaning teeth and visiting the dentist. Firstly, however, we look, as in the previous chapter, at the child's dental treatment history.

8.2 Treatment experience
We start by looking at the proportions of children who had never visited a dentist (Table 8.1) and see that there has been a decrease in this statistic between 1973 and 1983 particularly among the younger children, where the proportions who had never visited the dentist were higher than among the older children. Among five year olds, for example, the proportion of children who had never visited a dentist had halved between 1973 and 1983 (from 29% to 13%).

Improvements were evident in each of the social class groups but particularly among Social Classes III M and Social Classes IV and V, where among five year olds the proportion who had never visited the dentist decreased by over a half.

In terms of regional change, decreases were seen everywhere among the five year olds and this decrease was particularly large in the Midlands and East Anglia (from 37% to 13%) so that in 1983 there was no difference between the regions in terms of the proportion of five year olds who had never visited a dentist.

These changes, particularly among children from the Social Classes IV and V and among children from what had been the worst region in terms of the proportion of children who had never visited the dentist, are extremely encouraging. It is difficult to assess what has caused such large changes among these groups. It may be the result of an effort on behalf of the Community Dental Service to improve the dental health of the groups known to be in the least fortunate position. It is also the case that since 1973 there has been a very large increase in the amount of television advertising for toothpaste which puts across the message that children should visit the dentist and this must surely have had some effect.

It has been shown in previous chapters that the condition of children's teeth as measured by the dental examiner had improved greatly between 1973 and 1983 and this improvement is apparent in the change in children's treatment experiences over the whole of their lives so far.

Table 8.2 shows the very large increases in the proportion of children who had visited a dentist and had not had a filling or an extraction. Among five year olds, this figure had doubled from a quarter to a half. Among eight year olds, however, the improvements were more striking with a four-fold increase in the proportion of children with no fillings or extractions from 7% in 1973 to 28% in 1983.

Improvements were obvious in each social class group. Among the five year olds, those from Social Class III M had improved considerably while those from Social Classes IV and V had not made such large improvements and were left, despite an increase from 24% to 37%, in a comparatively poor position.

Among eight year olds, the increase in the proportion who had visited the dentist and not received fillings or had extractions was particularly striking among those from Social Classes IV and V where the figure was 2% in 1973 and 22% in 1983.

Table 8.1 Proportion of children who have never been to the dentist in England and Wales in 1973 and 1983, by social class and region

	Age (years)							
	5		8		12		14	15
	1973	1983	1973	1983	1973	1983	1973	1983
Social class								
I, II, III N	18%	10%	3%	3%	1%	1%	1%	–
III M	32%	15%	9%	4%	4%	3%	2%	1%
IV, V.	40%	17%	20%	10%	4%	2%	10%	1%
Region								
The North	30%	14%	9%	5%	5%	3%	4%	2%
Midlands and East Anglia	37%	13%	14%	4%	4%	2%	3%	–
Wales and the South West	23%	15%	4%	4%	3%	1%	3%	1%
London and the South East	26%	12%	8%	4%	2%	2%	4%	1%
England and Wales	29%	13%	9%	4%	3%	2%	3%	1%

For bases see Appendix A

Table 8.2 Proportion of children in England and Wales in 1973 and 1983 who had visited the dentist and had not had a filling or extraction, by social class and region

	Age (years)							
	5		8		12		14	15
	1973	1983	1973	1983	1973	1983	1973	1983
Social Class								
I, II, III N	38%	62%	10%	31%	3%	10%	3%	5%
III M	20%	53%	7%	24%	2%	6%	3%	3%
IV, V	24%	37%	2%	22%	1%	6%	2%	4%
Region								
The North	24%	52%	5%	20%	2%	6%	3%	2%
Midlands and East Anglia	22%	52%	5%	30%	1%	9%	3%	7%
Wales and the South West	25%	42%	11%	20%	3%	7%	2%	4%
London and the South East	31%	60%	9%	35%	2%	9%	3%	5%
England and Wales	26%	54%	7%	28%	3%	8%	3%	4%

For bases see Appendix A

Table 8.3 Proportion of children in England and Wales in 1973 and 1983 who had ever had an extraction by social class and region

	Age (years)							
	5		8		12		14	15
	1973	1983	1973	1983	1973	1983	1973	1983
Social Class								
I, II, III N	17%	7%	62%	36%	76%	64%	74%	65%
III M	28%	12%	66%	40%	82%	65%	80%	75%
IV, V	23%	15%	59%	46%	79%	68%	77%	73%
Region								
The North	28%	15%	73%	54%	81%	73%	81%	79%
Midlands and East Anglia	24%	10%	64%	37%	87%	63%	79%	65%
Wales and the South West	21%	12%	60%	47%	71%	69%	78%	74%
London and the South East	19%	4%	56%	25%	76%	58%	70%	64%
England and Wales	24%	10%	64%	39%	78%	65%	77%	70%

For bases see Appendix A

Table 8.4 Proportion of children in England and Wales in 1973 and 1983 who had ever had a filling, by social class and region

	Age (years)							
	5		8		12		14	15
	1973	1983	1973	1983	1973	1983	1973	1983
Social Class								
I, II, III N	38%	26%	74%	56%	89%	81%	93%	92%
III M	35%	27%	64%	63%	82%	82%	80%	90%
IV, V	22%	40%	56%	50%	82%	76%	71%	87%
Region								
The North	31%	24%	60%	56%	79%	79%	78%	90%
Midlands and East Anglia	29%	33%	54%	56%	81%	77%	79%	90%
Wales and the South West	39%	37%	71%	64%	85%	85%	85%	90%
London and the South East	40%	27%	74%	56%	90%	83%	88%	90%
England and Wales	34%	28%	65%	57%	84%	80%	83%	90%

For bases see Appendix A

The proportions of children who had ever had an extraction decreased in each of the age groups, in each of the social class groups and in each of the regions (Table 8.3). Among the five and eight year olds, the relative positions of children from Social Class III M and children from Social Classes IV and V changed between 1973 and 1983. In 1973 the former had a higher proportion with experience of extractions than the latter but the opposite was true in 1983. Children from Social Classes I, II and III N maintained the position of having the lowest experience of extractions.

Also among the five and eight year olds, those from the North retained the position of having the highest experience of extractions, despite large decreases over the ten years. Those from London and the South East showed the largest decreases in the proportion with experience of extraction, among five year olds in this region the proportion decreased from 19% to just 4%.

The changes over the ten years in the proportion of children who had ever had a filling (Table 8.4) are more difficult to interpret. A filling, although an indication of

Table 8.5   The proportion of children in England and Wales in 1973 and 1983 who had ever had gas at the dental surgery

| | Age (years) | | | | | | | |
| | 5 | | 8 | | 12 | | 14 | 15 |
	1973	1983	1973	1983	1973	1983	1973	1983
	%	%	%	%	%	%	%	%
Had gas	19	7	49	27	59	35	58	47
Had not	81	93	51	73	41	65	42	53
All children	100	100	100	100	100	100	100	100

For bases see Appendix A

past decay, is still preferable in dental terms to an extraction. Table 8.4 seems to indicate two opposite trends in the levels of fillings over the ten year period; a decrease, connected with the overall decrease in the level of dental disease and an increase, whereby diseased teeth were being filled rather than extracted.

Overall, among the younger children, there was a slight decrease in the proportion of children who had ever had a filling between 1973 and 1983. In Chapter 4 it was shown that the proportion of five year olds with some filled teeth was 26% in 1973 and 23% in 1983. These are slightly lower figures than those given by the parents when asked whether the five year olds had ever had a filling. However, as was said in the previous chapter this is largely accounted for by the fact that the survey measurement presented in Chapter 4 was a measure of teeth that were filled (otherwise sound). If we look at teeth that were recorded as filled (otherwise sound) and filled and decayed, we find that the parents of the five year olds were, perhaps not surprisingly, very accurate in their assessment of whether or not their child had had a filling.

Among five year olds, the proportion who had had a filling among those from Social Classes I, II, III N and III M decreased between 1973 and 1983 but among those from Social Classes IV and V, this proportion increased from 22% in 1973 to 40% in 1983. Among the regions, changes in the prevalence of fillings occurred only in the North (where the proportion decreased from 31% to 24%) and in London and the South East (where it decreased from 40% to 27%).

Among the eight year olds, there was a significant decrease in the proportion of those from Social Classes I, II, III N who had ever had a filling (from 74% in 1973 to 56% in 1983). There was a similar decrease in the proportion who had ever had a filling among the eight year olds from London and the South East.

Among the twelve year olds there was little change in the proportion of children who had ever had a filling while among the oldest children a slight increase in this proportion was apparent.

Table 8.5 shows the proportions of children in 1973 and 1983 who had ever had gas at the dentist's surgery. In 1973, by the age of eight, one half of the children had had gas. In 1983 this figure had considerably reduced. Among the eight year olds in 1983 27% had had gas.

Reductions in the proportions of children who had had gas were apparent in each of the age groups.

8.3 Dental care
In this section we look at two aspects of dental care, tooth brushing and visiting the dentist, to see how habits changed between 1973 and 1983.

It appears from Table 8.6 that the frequency with which children clean their teeth increased between 1973 and 1983, particularly among the youngest children. In 1973, 56% of five year olds were said to clean their teeth twice a day or more often while in 1983 this was said of 69% of the five year olds. Among the oldest children, however, there was no significant difference between the reported frequency of cleaning the teeth in 1973 and in 1983. It would seem that children growing up in this ten year period increased their frequency of tooth brushing. The fifteen year olds in 1983 brushed their teeth more frequently than the five year olds in 1973. There was already a higher proportion of five year olds in 1983 than in 1973 who brushed their teeth twice or more a day and if they behave over the next ten years as their counterparts in 1973 there will be a still higher proportion of fifteen year olds in 1993 who brush their teeth twice or more a day.

Children in 1983 also appear to visit the dentist at an earlier age than in 1973 (Table 8.7) and this was particularly true of the younger children. However, as was noted in the previous chapter, the results for the older children are likely to be less reliable than the results for the younger children because of the effect of memory. For the youngest children, a significantly higher proportion had visited the dentist aged three or less in 1983 (61%) than had been the case in 1973 (41%).

Similar improvements can be seen in the regularity with which the children visited the dentist (Table 8.8). In each of the age groups a significantly higher proportion of children were said to be regular attenders in 1983 than in 1973. Among eight year olds for example 51% were regular dental attenders in 1973 compared with 62% in 1983.

This increase in dental care in terms of tooth brushing and visiting the dentist is likely to have been connected with the improvement in dental health between 1973 and 1983. However, we know from Chapter 6 that among children with poorer dental habits there was still a substantial improvement in dental health as measured by the dental examination.

Table 8.6 Frequency of brushing the teeth among children in England and Wales in 1973 and 1983

Frequency of brushing the teeth	Age (years)							
	5		8		12		14	15
	1973	1983	1973	1983	1973	1983	1973	1983
	%	%	%	%	%	%	%	%
Three or more times a day	5	3	5	4	6	5	8	12
Twice a day	51	66	52	62	55	62	60	60
Once a day	33	27	33	27	31	25	24	21
Less than once a day	11	4	10	7	8	7	8	6
All frequencies	100	100	100	100	100	100	100	100

For bases see Appendix A

Table 8.7 Age first visited the dentist for children in England and Wales in 1973 and 1983

Age (years) at first visit	Current age (years)							
	5		8		12		14	15
	1973	1983	1973	1983	1973	1983	1973	1983
	%	%	%	%	%	%	%	%
Three or less	41	61	39	49	35	39	30	37
Four	18	19	18	19	16	20	17	19
Five or more	11	8	34	28	45	38	50	43
Never been	29	13	9	4	3	2	3	1
All children	100	100	100	100	100	100	100	100

For bases see Appendix A

Table 8.8 Attendance pattern among children in England and Wales in 1973 and 1983

Attendance pattern	Age							
	5		8		12		14	15
	1973	1983	1973	1983	1973	1983	1973	1983
	%	%	%	%	%	%	%	%
Regular attenders	39	57	51	62	53	64	48	59
Occasional attenders	8	19	10	14	15	14	19	21
Only with trouble	53	24	39	24	32	22	33	20
All attenders	100	100	100	100	100	100	100	100

For bases see Appendix A

8.4 Summary

In 1973 29% of five year olds in England and Wales had never been to the dentist but in 1983 this was so for only 13%. Children are also more likely to be visiting the dentist without needing either extractions or fillings. In 1973 a quarter of the five year olds had been to the dentist but needed no fillings or extractions, in 1983 the proportion was 54%. Even among the eight year olds there was a dramatic improvement. In 1973 7% of eight year olds had been to a dentist but needed no extractions or fillings, in 1983 the comparable propor-

tion was 28%. This improvement was to be seen in all the social class groups and all the regions of England and Wales. There was also a reduction in the proportions of children who had had gas at the dental surgery.

A higher proportion of parents said their children brushed their teeth twice a day or more in 1983 than had been the case in 1973, and a higher proportion said the children attended regularly for check-ups in 1983 than had been the case in 1973.

9 The periodontal condition of children

9.1 Introduction

Previous chapters have discussed the condition of children's teeth and shown that, while there was a large improvement here between 1973 and 1983, there was still considerable variation in the health of children's teeth between the constituent countries of the United Kingdom. A further indicator of dental health is the condition of the gums and it is this, the periodontal health of the children, that is discussed in this chapter.

When the first children's dental health survey was carried out, the dental examination included the measurement of three conditions associated with the condition of the gums. For each of the six segments of the mouth, the dentist recorded the presence of gum inflammation, the presence of any debris and the presence of calculus. In order to retain comparability with this previous study, the dental examination in 1983 was designed to reproduce identically these assessments.

However, since the 1973 survey, new ways of assessing such problems have been developed. One method that has been used in other studies involves the assessment of pocketing and gingivitis by the use of a probe as specified by the World Health Organisation (WHO)* and it was decided that this method would be incorporated into the 1983 survey examination. The use of this probe to assess gingivitis can elicit bleeding and, therefore, it was important to ensure that there was no possibility of the dental examiner spreading infection from one child to another. To eliminate any risk it was decided that a separate sterilised probe should be used for each child. This decision meant that the cost of making the assessment with the probe on all the children in all the age groups would be prohibitive and it was therefore decided that probes should be used to assess pocketing and gingivitis on the children amongst whom adverse periodontal conditions were likely to be most prevalent, that is the fifteen year olds.

When the results from the dental examinations were first available for analysis we carried out tests to see if there was any association between the field work findings and the variability measured in the calibration tests carried out during the training period. It was found that, as indeed it has been found on previous studies, the data about gum condition using the 1973 criteria were subject to variation which related to the individual dentist who performed the examination.

Reference to the calibration results showed that members of certain teams of dentists who trained together tended to assess the condition of the gums in a similar way to others in their team but in a different way to other teams. As dentists who trained together worked in the same part of the United Kingdom for the survey, we have certain reservations about these gum assessments when we come to look at them for the separate countries of the United Kingdom.

We have more confidence in the results gained by the use of the periodontal probe because this is a more objective measurement whereas the 1973 criteria relied more on the dentist's opinion. We unfortunately, however, only have the measurements using this probe for the fifteen year olds. We therefore present the results on periodontal problems using both the visual assessment and the periodontal probe but alert readers to certain reservations we have concerning the former.

9.2 The visual assessment of the gums

The condition of the gums was assessed for children in each age group using the same criteria as that used in the 1973 survey. The six segments of the mouth were examined separately and the presence of gum inflammation, calculus and debris were recorded.

Table 9.1 shows the proportion of children with some gum inflammation. It can be seen that the proportion of children recorded as having some inflammation increased with age from 19% among five year olds to 46% among the eight year olds. Among the older children the proportion with some inflammation varied little with age, with about one half of all children being recorded as having gum inflammation. Again, it must be stressed that one must be wary of making regional comparisons of these data due to the examiner-variability associated with them.

The proportion of children recorded with some calculus increased with age throughout the age range five to fifteen (Table 9.2). Among five year olds, 3% were recorded with some calculus, this proportion rose to 16% of the ten year olds and to 33% of the fifteen year olds.

The third condition measured during the examination was the presence of debris, such as plaque, around the teeth. Table 9.3 shows that in the age range seven to fifteen one half of the children seen had some debris.

In terms, then, of these assessments of the condition of the gums, we find a rather unsatisfactory picture of the periodontal health of children. Among the oldest

---

* For a description of this probe and its use in assessment see the dental criteria in Appendix C.

Table 9.1 The proportion of children with some gum inflammation

	Age (years)										
	5	6	7	8	9	10	11	12	13	14	15
England	19%	27%	40%	48%	52%	51%	55%	51%	52%	51%	50%
Wales	11%	14%	31%	38%	39%	31%	46%	43%	38%	34%	30%
Scotland	20%	17%	29%	32%	32%	31%	34%	37%	34%	37%	33%
Northern Ireland	20%	31%	58%	53%	56%	58%	66%	55%	58%	56%	52%
United Kingdom	19%	26%	39%	46%	50%	49%	53%	49%	50%	49%	48%

For bases see Appendix A

Table 9.2 The proportion of children with some calculus

	Age (years)										
	5	6	7	8	9	10	11	12	13	14	15
England	4%	4%	9%	13%	15%	16%	21%	21%	24%	27%	34%
Wales	1%	2%	5%	8%	13%	18%	17%	18%	24%	20%	26%
Scotland	2%	4%	7%	8%	14%	17%	20%	21%	21%	25%	29%
Northern Ireland	–	2%	7%	11%	16%	21%	21%	28%	30%	33%	38%
United Kingdom	3%	4%	8%	13%	15%	16%	20%	21%	24%	26%	33%

For bases see Appendix A

Table 9.3 The proportion of children with some debris

	Age (years)										
	5	6	7	8	9	10	11	12	13	14	15
England	29%	36%	51%	56%	57%	57%	57%	49%	49%	50%	49%
Wales	17%	30%	41%	52%	52%	42%	48%	40%	36%	32%	32%
Scotland	29%	33%	48%	53%	53%	51%	49%	42%	40%	43%	39%
Northern Ireland	27%	39%	56%	54%	57%	60%	61%	49%	53%	53%	47%
United Kingdom	29%	36%	50%	55%	56%	56%	56%	48%	48%	49%	47%

For bases see Appendix A

Table 9.4 The proportions of children with gum inflammation, calculus and debris in England and Wales in 1973 and 1983

Age (years)	Gum inflammation		Calculus		Debris	
	1973	1983	1973	1983	1973	1983
5	26%	18%	5%	3%	39%	29%
6	35%	26%	5%	4%	48%	36%
7	50%	40%	9%	9%	62%	50%
8	56%	47%	15%	13%	67%	55%
9	56%	51%	17%	15%	67%	56%
10	56%	50%	21%	16%	65%	56%
11	59%	54%	26%	20%	65%	56%
12	57%	50%	28%	21%	64%	49%
13	55%	51%	31%	24%	59%	48%
14	54%	50%	33%	26%	56%	49%
15	51%	49%	34%	33%	51%	47%

For bases see Appendix A

children one half had gum inflammation, one third had calculus and a half had some debris around the teeth.

As noted in the previous section these visual measures of gum condition were retained in the 1983 examination in order to give comparable data to that collected in 1973. In Table 9.4 the results for the two surveys are presented. It can be seen that, in the case of gum inflammation, there appeared to be a slightly lower proportion of children with this condition in 1983 than there had been in 1973, most noticeably among the younger children. For example, in 1973, 35% of six year olds in England and Wales had some inflammation compared with 26% of six year olds in 1983.

The proportion of children aged between ten and fourteen with some calculus had also appeared to decrease. For example among twelve year olds 28% had some calculus in 1973 compared with 21% in 1983. The proportions of children with calculus had not, however, changed over the ten years among the younger or, indeed, the oldest children.

Of the three conditions assessed the one that showed the most change over the ten year period was the presence of debris. There had been a decrease in the proportion of children with debris in all the age groups. Among nine year olds, for example, the proportion decreased from 67% in 1973 to 56% in 1983.

Although the results suggested that there have been improvements in the health of children's gums over the ten year period these improvements are not as large as the improvements found in the health of children's teeth shown in the previous chapters.

9.3 Pocketing and gingivitis among fifteen year olds

The presence of pocketing and gingivitis was assessed on the fifteen year olds with the aid of the WHO periodontal probe. This probe was inserted into the sulcus on six nominated teeth and run along the surface of the tooth. A measurement was taken as to the depth of the sulcus at its deepest part according to whether it was under 3.5 mm (no pocketing) between 3.5 mm and 5.5 mm (mild pocketing) or over 5.5 mm (severe pocketing). If the action of running the probe along the pocket elicited bleeding then the child was judged to have gingivitis.

Table 9.5 shows the proportions of fifteen year olds with pocketing and gingivitis assessed in this manner. The measure of pocketing is not shown separately for mild and severe pocketing because, in fact, less than half of one per cent of the children had the more severe condition. Overall 9% of fifteen year old children in the United Kingdom had some pocketing and there were no significant differences between the proportions of children with pocketing in the constituent countries of the United Kingdom.

The proportion of children with gingivitis as measured by the probe was much higher than the proportion with pocketing; 48% of fifteen year olds in the United Kingdom had some gingivitis. There was a significantly higher proportion of fifteen year olds in Scotland and Northern Ireland with gingivitis than in England or Wales.

Table 9.5 also shows that the presence of pocketing and gingivitis are related. In the United Kingdom 7% of fifteen year olds had both pocketing and gingivitis and thus just 2% of fifteen year olds had pocketing without associated gingivitis.

Table 9.6 shows the distribution around the mouth of pocketing and gingivitis as measured by the probe. In the case of pocketing, such a comparatively small proportion was recorded in each segment one can draw no firm conclusions as to how it was distributed around the mouth. In the case of gingivitis there was a difference between the proportions of fifteen year olds with gingivitis in the individual segments. The proportion of children with gingivitis in the posterior segments of the mouth was higher than the proportion with gingivitis in the anterior segments of the mouth. For example, 20% of fifteen year olds had gingivitis in the upper right posterior segment compared with 9% with gingivitis in their upper anterior segment. A higher proportion of fifteen year olds had gingivitis in their lower posterior mouth segments than in the upper posterior mouth segments. For example, 30% of fifteen year olds had gingivitis in the lower left posterior segment compared with 13% who had gingivitis in their upper left posterior segment.

Table 9.5 The proportion of fifteen year olds with pocketing and gingivitis among fifteen year olds

	Proportion with:		
	Pocketing	Gingivitis	Pocketing and gingivitis
England	9%	47%	7%
Wales	9%	41%	7%
Scotland	7%	56%	6%
Northern Ireland	11%	60%	10%
United Kingdom	9%	48%	7%

For bases see Appendix A

Table 9.6 The presence of pocketing and gingivitis among fifteen year olds by mouth segment

	Upper left	Upper middle	Upper right	Lower right	Lower middle	Lower left	Any mouth segment
Proportion of fifteen year olds with:							
Some pocketing	1%	1%	2%	3%	–	4%	9%
Some gingivitis	13%	9%	20%	24%	6%	30%	48%

For bases see Appendix A

Table 9.7 Proportion of fifteen year olds with pocketing, gingivitis and active decay

	Proportion of fifteen year olds:			
	With pocketing	Without pocketing	With gingivitis	Without gingivitis
	%	%	%	%
Some active decay	57	40	42	41
No active decay	43	60	58	59
All fifteen year olds	100	100	100	100
Base	92	996	518	570

Table 9.7 shows the relationship between pocketing and gingivitis in fifteen year olds, and dental decay. It can be seen that a higher proportion of children with pocketing than without had some actively decayed teeth. Of children with pocketing, 57% had some active decay compared with 40% of children with no pocketing. There was however no noticeable association between the presence of gingivitis and the presence of dental decay.

Finally we look in Table 9.8 at the relationship between gum disease in the fifteen year olds and household social class. This table shows that there were no statistically significant differences between children from different social classes in the proportion of children with either pocketing or gingivitis.

So it can be seen that at the age of fifteen about a half of all children have gingivitis and that, unlike the situation with regard to the health of the teeth, there was little difference between children in the different social class groups in terms of the health of the gums.

9.4 Summary

Assessments were made on the condition of the children's gums using the same criteria as in 1973. This assessment is not a totally objective measure and is subject to some examiner-variability which restrict the amount of detailed analysis that is tenable. In addition to repeating the earlier assessment a new assessment was used based on the WHO method of assessing the periodontal condition. This method was found to have less variability but could only be carried out on a small sample of children, (fifteen year olds only), because of the high cost of supplying sterile probes for the examination.

There was some suggestion that children's mouths tended to be cleaner in 1983 than 1973 (there were lower proportions of children with debris) but in terms of inflammation there was no apparent improvement over ten years comparable to that seen with respect to decay.

Table 9.8 Pocketing, gingivitis and social class of household

Social class of household	Proportion of fifteen year olds with:		
	Pocketing	Gingivitis	Pocketing and gingivitis
England			
I, II, III N	8%	47%	7%
III M	9%	51%	7%
IV, V	9%	42%	8%
All	9%	47%	7%
Wales			
I, II, III N	7%	42%	6%
III M	10%	37%	7%
IV, V	8%	53%	6%
All	9%	41%	7%
Scotland			
I, II, III N	10%	52%	8%
III M	7%	53%	5%
IV, V	6%	60%	4%
All	7%	56%	6%
Northern Ireland			
I, II, III N	16%	60%	14%
III M	6%	62%	5%
IV, V	14%	57%	14%
All	11%	60%	10%
United Kingdom			
I, II, III N	8%	47%	7%
III M	9%	49%	7%
IV, V	9%	44%	8%
All	9%	48%	7%

For bases see Appendix A

10 The orthodontic condition of children

10.1 Introduction

In addition to the information collected about the health of children's teeth and gums, the survey dental examination also gathered information on various occlusal features and on the prevalence of, and need for, orthodontic treatment.

The majority of assessments concerned the occlusion of the permanent incisors and it was therefore decided that the section of the examination that involved orthodontic assessments should only be carried out if a child had at least one permanent upper incisor present.

Assessments were made on the size of the child's overjet, whether the incisors were rotated, instanding or in an edge-to-edge relationship, whether an increased overbite had caused traumatic injury and whether or not the child's teeth were crowded. The dentist also recorded whether or not the child had received orthodontic treatment in the past and whether, in the dentist's opinion, the child needed or would need orthodontic treatment (or referral to an orthodontist for an assessment of treatment need).

Table 10.1 shows the proportions of children who were assessed as having at least one of the following conditions: an overjet of 5mm or more, an incisor that was rotated, instanding or in an edge-to-edge relationship, traumatic injury due to an increased overbite,

or crowding of the teeth. It can be seen that among children for whom a survey orthodontic assessment was made, a high proportion had at least one of the conditions assessed. We look in more detail at the different orthodontic assessments later in the chapter.

Table 10.2 shows the proportions of children who were receiving or who had received orthodontic treatment. The information concerning orthodontic treatment was collected at two points during the dental examination. First, during the assessment of the children's teeth, the dentist recorded whether or not a child had had any orthodontic extractions. Second, during the orthodontic assessment, the dentist recorded whether the child was wearing, or had worn, an orthodontic appliance. The proportion of children currently wearing an appliance was highest among the twelve and thirteen year olds while, not surprisingly, the proportion of children who had ever had orthodontic treatment was highest among the oldest children. Among the oldest children a third had received or were currently receiving orthodontic treatment. It can be seen that, of the different types of treatment children receive, appliance therapy without orthodontic extractions was the least common while the proportions of children who had had treatment in the form of orthodontic extractions alone and the proportions who had had orthodontic extractions and appliance therapy were similar.

Table 10.1 The presence of orthodontic conditions included in the survey assessment

	Age (years)										
	5	6	7	8	9	10	11	12	13	14	15
	%	%	%	%	%	%	%	%	%	%	%
Has at least one anomaly	1	20	58	78	79	77	76	71	73	70	73
Has not	2	10	22	20	20	23	24	29	27	30	27
Not assessed	97	70	20	2	1	–	–	–	–	–	–
Total	100	100	100	100	100	100	100	100	100	100	100

For bases see Appendix A

Table 10.2 Experience of orthodontic treatment among children

	Age (years)										
	5	6	7	8	9	10	11	12	13	14	15
	%	%	%	%	%	%	%	%	%	%	%
Under treatment now	–	–	–	–	1	1	3	9	8	6	5
Had treatment											
Extractions only	–	–	1	–	1	1	4	5	7	9	12
Appliance only	–	–	–	1	1	3	3	2	4	4	5
Extractions and											
appliance	–	–	–	–	–	1	1	3	6	10	12
Never had treatment	3	30	79	97	97	94	89	81	75	71	66
Not assessed	97	70	20	2	–	–	–	–	–	–	–
Total	100	100	100	100	100	100	100	100	100	100	100

For bases see Appendix A

Table 10.3 The proportion of children who were in need of orthodontic treatment by whether or not treatment had been received in the past

	Age (years)										
	5	6	7	8	9	10	11	12	13	14	15
	%	%	%	%	%	%	%	%	%	%	%
Not assessed	97	70	20	2	–	–	–	–	–	–	–
Needs no orthodontic treatment	2	20	40	42	42	43	46	45	47	47	45
Has had treatment in past and:											
Needs further treatment	–	–	–	1	1	2	4	4	7	7	10
Needs no treatment now	–	–	–	–	1	3	4	6	11	15	20
Needs treatment and has had none in past	1	9	40	55	55	50	43	36	27	25	20
Under treatment now	–	–	–	–	1	2	3	9	8	6	5
Total	100	100	100	100	100	100	100	100	100	100	100

For bases see Appendix A

Although we know whether or not a child had received orthodontic treatment the survey did not provide information as to the orthodontic state for which the treatment was provided. We can look however generally at the relationship between whether or not the children had previously had orthodontic treatment and whether they needed orthodontic treatment or assessment for treatment. The need for orthodontic treatment was assessed by the dentist on all children who were not currently undergoing treatment. It was a subjective judgement and did not necessarily relate directly to the assessment the dentist had made on the orthodontic conditions assessed for the survey. For example, the dentist could have recorded a child as having overcrowding on the survey criteria but felt there was not a need for treatment.

Table 10.3 shows that among children in the age groups up to thirteen, those who had some treatment in the past were fairly evenly divided between those who did not now, in the survey dental examiners opinion, need orthodontic treatment at the time of the examination and those that did.

In the older ages, the majority of those who had received orthodontic treatment in the past were not in need of orthodontic treatment at the time of the survey.

Little orthodontic treatment is carried out before children are ten years old and the survey shows that among the younger children more have potential or actual orthodontic treatment need than do not. From the age at which treatment is provided the picture among those who have never had treatment changes, with those who do not need treatment outnumbering those who do. This change is clearly affected by the fact that orthodontic treatment is provided for some 30% of children by the time they are fifteen years old. It may also be affected by the natural process of growth and development of the child. Although the proportion of children needing orthodontic treatment who have never had such treatment decreases over the age groups ten to fifteen it is still as high as a quarter of fourteen year olds and a fifth of fifteen year olds.

The need for orthodontic treatment and the provision of orthodontic treatment is discussed in more detail later in this chapter. The following sections show the survey results for the individual items included in the survey orthodontic assessment.

10.2 The occlusion of the incisors

Overjet

The measurement of overjet is the horizontal distance from the front edge of the upper incisors to the front edge of the lower incisors, measured when the teeth are in natural occlusion.

Table 10.4 shows the measurement of overjet on the upper left permanent incisors. (This measurement was also made on the upper right incisor but, as the distributions of measurements were very similar to those for the upper left incisor, we present information on the latter measure only.)

It can be seen from the table that among the youngest age groups this measurement was not assessed on the vast majority of children due to the fact that the permanent upper incisors had not yet erupted. Among the older children there were no large differences between age groups in the distribution of measures of overjet, although there was a lower proportion of the older children with an overjet of 5mm or more compared with children in the middle of the age range. For example, 15% of fourteen year olds had an overjet of 5mm or more compared with 24% of the eight year olds.

Table 10.5 shows how the presence of an overjet of 5mm or more is related to the presence of at least one other of the orthodontic anomalies. (The other measured anomalies were the presence of rotated, instanding or edge-to-edge incisors, gingival damage associated with a deep overbite, and crowding.) It can be seen that in each of the age groups the majority of children who had an increased overjet also had one of the other measured orthodontic anomalies and less than one in ten had an overjet of 5mm or more and no other orthodontic anomaly.

Table 10.4 Proportions of children with different measures of overjet on the upper left permanent incisor

Measure of overjet	Age (years)										
	5	6	7	8	9	10	11	12	13	14	15
	%	%	%	%	%	%	%	%	%	%	%
Negative or zero	–	1	3	3	3	3	3	3	4	4	5
Positive less than 5mm	2	15	49	67	72	74	76	75	78	81	78
5mm but less than 7mm	–	3	12	16	13	13	14	13	11	10	11
7mm or more	–	1	5	8	9	9	8	8	7	5	4
Not assessed	98	80	31	6	2	–	1	1	1	–	1
Total	100	100	100	100	100	100	100	100	100	100	100

For bases see Appendix A

Table 10.5 Proportion of children with an increased overjet and any other orthodontic anomaly

	Age (years)										
	5	6	7	8	9	10	11	12	13	14	15
	%	%	%	%	%	%	%	%	%	%	%
Had overjet of 5mm or more only	–	1	5	9	8	8	7	7	6	5	4
Had overjet of 5mm or more and other anomaly	1	3	12	15	13	15	14	14	11	10	11
Had other anomaly	–	6	30	50	57	54	55	50	56	55	57
Had no anomaly	1	10	22	20	20	23	24	29	27	30	27
Not assessed	98	80	31	6	2	–	1	1	1	–	1
Total	100	100	100	100	100	100	100	100	100	100	100

For bases see Appendix A

Instanding incisors

In addition to measuring the size of the children's overjet other assessments were made concerning the occlusion of the permanent incisors. These included the presence of incisors that were instanding, that is where an upper incisor rests behind the lower incisors when the teeth are in occlusion, the presence of incisors that were edge-to-edge, that is, where the edge of an upper incisor rests on the edge of a lower incisor when the teeth are in occlusion, the presence of upper incisors rotated through an angle of 30 degrees or more and the presence of traumatic overbite, that is, damage to the gums in the anterior sections of the mouth associated with increased overbite.

Table 10.6 shows the proportions of children with instanding permanent central or lateral incisors. It can be seen that only a very small proportion of children had an instanding central incisor and a slightly higher proportion had a lateral incisor instanding.

Among children age nine and over there were no statistically significant differences between children of different ages in the proportions of children with at least one instanding incisor. Very few children were assessed as having an instanding incisor in the absence of the other measured orthodontic anomalies (Table 10.7).

Edge-to-edge incisors

Table 10.8 shows the proportions of children with edge-to-edge incisors. As with instanding incisors, it can be seen that in the majority of age groups, a higher proportion of children had lateral incisors rather than central incisors that were edge-to-edge. Overall, the highest proportions of children with at least one edge-to-edge incisor, were found among the older children. For example, 9% of fifteen year olds had an edge-to-edge incisor compared with 5% of nine year olds.

As with the case of instanding incisors very few children had an edge-to-edge incisor alone without any of the other orthodontic anomalies (Table 10.9).

Rotated incisors

Table 10.10 shows that the proportions of children in each of the age groups with a permanent incisor rotated through an angle of 30 degrees or more were small (less than one in ten) and that none of the sampled children had a rotated incisor without having one of the other measured orthodontic anomalies.

Traumatic overbite

Traumatic injury caused by a deep overbite was found among very few children in the United Kingdom and as was the case with rotated incisors it was not found without one of the other measured anomalies (Table 10.11).

10.3 Crowding

The most common developmental anomaly seen among children was crowding of the teeth. A child was defined as having a crowded mouth if there was insufficient space in the mouth to accommodate the teeth without crowding or overlap. As with the other orthodontic assessments, the examination for crowding was made only if at least one of the permanent upper incisors was present. From Table 10.12 it can be seen that, from the age of eight, in each age group, over 60% of children in the United Kingdom had a crowded mouth and that the highest proportion was found among children in the age range eight to eleven.

Table 10.6 The proportion of children with one or more permanent incisors instanding

	Age (years)										
	5	6	7	8	9	10	11	12	13	14	15
Proportion of children with one or more:											
Central incisors instanding	–	1%	2%	2%	2%	2%	2%	2%	1%	1%	1%
Lateral incisors instanding	–	–	1%	4%	5%	6%	7%	6%	4%	5%	5%
Any incisors instanding	–	1%	3%	4%	7%	7%	7%	6%	6%	5%	5%

For bases see Appendix A

Table 10.7 Proportion of children with at least one instanding incisor or any other orthodontic anomaly

	Age (years)										
	5	6	7	8	9	10	11	12	13	14	15
	%	%	%	%	%	%	%	%	%	%	%
Had instanding incisor only	–	–	–	–	1	–	1	–	1	1	1
Had instanding incisor and other anomaly	–	1	3	4	6	7	6	6	5	4	4
Had other anomaly	1	19	55	74	72	70	69	65	67	65	68
Had no anomaly	2	10	22	20	20	23	24	29	27	30	27
Not assessed	97	70	20	2	1	–	–	–	–	–	–
Total	100	100	100	100	100	100	100	100	100	100	100

For bases see Appendix A

Table 10.8 The proportion of children with one or more edge-to-edge permanent incisors

	Age (years)										
	5	6	7	8	9	10	11	12	13	14	15
Proportion of children with one or more:											
Central incisors edge-to-edge	–	1%	2%	2%	2%	2%	2%	2%	2%	2%	4%
Lateral incisors edge-to-edge	–	–	1%	2%	4%	6%	4%	4%	6%	5%	8%
Any incisors edge-to-edge	–	1%	3%	5%	5%	7%	5%	5%	7%	8%	9%

For bases see Appendix A

Table 10.9 Proportion of children with at least one edge-to-edge incisor and any other orthodontic anomaly

	Age (years)										
	5	6	7	8	9	10	11	12	13	14	15
	%	%	%	%	%	%	%	%	%	%	%
Had edge-to-edge incisor only	–	–	1	1	1	1	1	1	2	3	2
Had edge-to-edge incisor and other anomaly	–	1	2	4	4	6	4	4	5	5	7
Had other anomaly	1	19	55	73	74	70	70	67	65	63	63
Had no anomaly	2	10	22	20	20	23	24	29	27	30	27
Not assessed	97	70	20	2	1	–	–	–	–	–	–
Total	100	100	100	100	100	100	100	100	100	100	100

For bases see Appendix A

A higher proportion of children in each of the age groups had crowded teeth and none of the other measured anomalies, than had crowded teeth and another of the anomalies. The table also shows that there was only a small proportion of children who had one of the measured anomalies without also having crowded teeth.

A further way of looking at the relationship between crowding and orthodontic treatment is to look at how the presence of crowded teeth is related to orthodontic extractions. Table 10.13 shows the proportion of children in the United Kingdom who had crowded teeth separately for crowding in the upper jaw and crowding in the lower jaw. Children aged five to seven have been omitted from this table due to the relatively large proportions of these age groups where an assessment was not made.

It can be seen that, up to the age of twelve, there is very little difference between the levels of crowding in the two jaws but that in the older age groups a higher proportion of children had crowding in their lower jaw than in their upper jaw. The proportion of children

with crowding in their upper jaw decreased with age up until the age of fourteen while fourteen and fifteen year olds had similar levels of crowding. The proportion of children with crowding in their lower jaw, decreased up to the age of twelve, and twelve, thirteen, fourteen and fifteen year olds had similar levels of crowding in that jaw.

Table 10.14 shows an interesting relationship between crowding and orthodontic extractions. The proportion of children who had no crowding in their upper jaw and had no orthodontic extractions varies very little between the age groups. The lower proportions of children with crowding in this jaw among the older children is due to the higher proportion of older children who have an uncrowded upper jaw but who have had orthodontic extractions, presumably to correct past crowding, or abnormal overjet.

In the lower jaw, there was less evidence of orthodontic extractions than in the upper jaw. In the age groups thirteen to fifteen a higher proportion of children had crowding and no orthodontic extractions in their lower jaw than in the upper jaw.

Table 10.10 The proportions of children with a rotated incisor and any other orthodontic anomaly

	Age (years)										
	5	6	7	8	9	10	11	12	13	14	15
	%	%	%	%	%	%	%	%	%	%	%
Had rotated incisor only	–	–	–	–	–	–	–	–	–	–	–
Had rotated incisor and other anomaly	–	1	6	8	8	5	4	4	4	4	5
Had other anomaly	1	19	52	70	71	72	71	68	67	65	68
Had no anomaly	2	10	22	20	20	23	25	28	28	30	27
Not assessed	97	70	20	2	1	–	–	–	–	–	–
Total	100	100	100	100	100	100	100	100	100	100	100

For bases see Appendix A

Table 10.11 The proportions of children with a traumatic overbite and any other orthodontic anomaly

	Age (years)										
	5	6	7	8	9	10	11	12	13	14	15
	%	%	%	%	%	%	%	%	%	%	%
Had traumatic overbite only	–	–	–	–	–	–	–	–	–	–	–
Had traumatic overbite and other anomaly	–	–	2	2	2	2	1	1	1	1	1
Had other anomaly	1	20	56	76	77	75	73	70	70	68	72
Had no anomaly	2	10	22	20	20	23	25	28	28	30	27
Not assessed	97	70	20	2	1	–	–	–	–	–	–
Total	100	100	100	100	100	100	100	100	100	100	100

For bases see Appendix A

Table 10.12 The proportions of children with crowding and any other anomaly

	Age (years)										
	5	6	7	8	9	10	11	12	13	14	15
	%	%	%	%	%	%	%	%	%	%	%
Had crowding only	1	11	32	42	42	38	43	38	41	41	40
Had crowding and other anomaly	–	7	21	26	27	29	23	24	21	20	24
Had other anomaly	–	2	5	10	10	10	9	10	10	9	9
Had no anomaly	2	10	22	20	20	23	24	29	27	30	27
Not assessed	97	70	20	2	1	–	–	–	–	–	–
Total	100	100	100	100	100	100	100	100	100	100	100

For bases see Appendix A

Table 10.13 The proportion of children with crowding in the upper and lower jaw

	Age (years)							
	8	9	10	11	12	13	14	15
	%	%	%	%	%	%	%	%
Upper jaw								
Crowding	55	59	54	50	47	46	41	42
No crowding	43	41	46	50	53	55	59	58
Not assessed	2	1	–	–	–	–	–	–
Total	100	100	100	100	100	100	100	100
Lower jaw								
Crowding	56	56	54	51	47	50	49	51
No crowding	41	43	46	49	52	51	51	49
Not assessed	2	1	–	–	–	–	–	–
Total	100	100	100	100	100	100	100	100

For bases see Appendix A

Table 10.14 Crowding and orthodontic extractions

	Age (years)							
	8	9	10	11	12	13	14	15
	%	%	%	%	%	%	%	%
Upper jaw								
Not crowded no extractions	43	41	45	46	44	44	44	42
Not assessed	2	1	–	–	–	–	–	–
Not crowded now had had some extractions	–	–	1	4	9	11	15	16
Crowded now, had had some extractions	–	–	1	2	5	6	6	8
Crowded now no extractions	55	59	53	48	42	40	35	34
Total	100	100	100	100	100	100	100	100
Lower jaw								
Not crowded no extractions	41	43	45	46	46	41	41	38
Not assessed	2	1	–	–	–	–	–	–
Not crowded now, had had some extractions	–	–	1	3	6	10	10	11
Crowded now, had had some extractions	–	–	–	1	3	4	5	6
Crowded now, no extractions	56	56	54	50	44	46	44	45
Total	100	100	100	100	100	100	100	100

For bases see Appendix A

10.4 Crowding and incisor problems

In this section we look at how some of the orthodontic assessments are related by looking at the variation between the presence of certain orthodontic measures among children with crowding and without.

Table 10.15 shows according to whether their teeth were crowded or not the proportion of children with the two extremes of the overjet measure; that is a zero or negative overjet measurement or a measurement of 5mm or more. There appears to be no relationship between a negative or zero overjet and crowding. There is also no significant difference in the proportion of children with a large overjet between those children with crowding and those without.

Table 10.15 Crowding and the extremes of overjet measure

Age (years)	Proportion with negative or zero overjet among those with:				Proportion with overjet of 5mm or more among those with:			
	No crowding		Some crowding		No crowding		Some crowding	
5	–	796	*	8	–	796	*	8
6	–	716	6%	147	1%	716	12%	147
7	2%	435	6%	488	11%	435	23%	488
8	3%	310	4%	658	19%	310	24%	658
9	3%	329	3%	732	19%	329	25%	732
10	3%	380	4%	772	21%	380	22%	772
11	3%	405	3%	769	18%	405	21%	769
12	3%	443	3%	722	18%	443	21%	722
13	3%	453	3%	739	16%	453	16%	739
14	2%	487	5%	761	13%	487	16%	761
15	6%	416	5%	740	11%	416	17%	740

Proportions not given for bases under 30

Table 10.16 shows the proportions of children with at least one instanding or edge-to-edge incisor among children with some crowding and among children with no crowding. It is not surprising to see that crowding of the teeth is related to the presence of instanding or edge-to-edge incisors. Among children aged nine and over there were proportionately about twice as many children with some instanding or edge-to-edge incisors among children with crowded teeth than among children with no crowding.

Table 10.16 Crowding and incisor relationship

Age (years)	Proportion with some instanding or edge-to-edge incisors among those with:			
	No crowding		Some crowding	
5	–	796	*	8
6	1%	716	6%	147
7	2%	435	9%	488
8	6%	310	10%	658
9	6%	329	12%	732
10	6%	380	15%	772
11	6%	405	12%	769
12	5%	443	13%	722
13	8%	453	13%	739
14	5%	487	13%	761
15	8%	416	16%	740

Proportions not given for bases under 30

10.5 National variation in the assessed orthodontic features

In this section we look at how the presence of orthodontic anomalies varied between the countries of the United Kingdom. In Table 10.17 we look at the proportion of children who had any of the following orthodontic features; an overjet of 5mm or more, an incisor that was rotated, instanding or in an edge-to-edge relationship, traumatic injury due to an increased overbite, or crowding of the teeth.

It can be seen that generally there was a lower proportion of children with at least one of these anomalies in Scotland than in England. Among thirteen year olds there was also a significantly lower proportion of children in Northern Ireland than in England with one of the measured anomalies and among fifteen year olds there was also a comparatively low proportion of children from Wales with any of the measured anomalies.

Table 10.18 shows the variation between the countries in the proportion of children with an overjet measurement of 5mm or more. Among the younger children it

can be seen that a higher proportion of children from England had a large overjet. For example among seven year olds, 20% from England had an overjet of 5mm or more compared with 6% from Wales, 14% from Scotland and 10% from Northern Ireland. Among the ten year olds, thirteen year olds and fourteen year olds there was a comparatively small proportion of children from Northern Ireland with an overjet measurement of 5mm or more while among the fifteen year olds, it was those from Wales who had the lowest proportion with an overjet of 5mm or more.

There was no significant national variation in the proportions of children with instanding incisors (Table 10.19) and there were few significant differences between the countries in the proportion of children with an edge-to-edge incisor. However, in the latter case, there was a significantly lower proportion of nine, ten, thirteen and fourteen year olds from Wales with one or more edge-to-edge incisors compared with children of those ages in England (Table 10.20).

There was considerable variation between the countries in the proportions of children with a rotated incisor (Table 10.21). Over the majority of age groups, Wales and Northern Ireland had significantly higher proportions of children with this feature than England and Scotland and, generally, Scotland had the lowest proportions of all the four countries.

As we have seen the prevalence of traumatic overbite was very small and Table 10.22 shows that there were few significant differences between the proportions of children with traumatic overbite in the constituent countries of the United Kingdom. There were indications, however, that Scotland had the lowest proportion of children with this condition and Northern Ireland the highest.

Table 10.23 shows the proportions of children from the different countries with crowded teeth. It can be seen that, except among the oldest children, there was very little difference between the proportions of children in Wales with crowding and the proportions in England. Generally, over the majority of ages, there were lower proportions with crowding among children in Scotland than among children in England and among children aged eleven to fourteen there were lower proportions of children in Northern Ireland with crowding than in England or Wales.

Table 10.17 The proportion of children with some orthodontic anomaly by country

	Age (years)										
	5	6	7	8	9	10	11	12	13	14	15
England	1%	18%	64%	77%	81%	77%	76%	73%	74%	71%	75%
Wales	1%	22%	62%	71%	79%	77%	76%	74%	72%	66%	63%
Scotland	1%	13%	60%	79%	75%	74%	69%	71%	66%	65%	64%
Northern Ireland	2%	18%	61%	79%	75%	82%	72%	71%	66%	66%	72%
United Kingdom	1%	17%	63%	78%	79%	77%	76%	71%	73%	70%	73%

For bases see Appendix A

Table 10.18   The proportion of children with an overjet measurement of 5mm or more by country

	Age (years)										
	5	6	7	8	9	10	11	12	13	14	15
England	–	4%	20%	24%	22%	22%	22%	21%	17%	15%	17%
Wales	1%	2%	6%	19%	22%	23%	18%	17%	19%	15%	10%
Scotland	–	3%	14%	20%	20%	21%	20%	22%	18%	15%	15%
Northern Ireland	–	2%	10%	15%	21%	16%	18%	18%	13%	10%	16%
United Kingdom	–	4%	17%	24%	21%	21%	22%	21%	18%	15%	15%

For bases see Appendix A

Table 10.19   The proportion of children with one or more permanent incisors instanding by country

	Age (years)										
	5	6	7	8	9	10	11	12	13	14	15
Proportion with one or more central incisors instanding											
England	–	1%	2%	2%	2%	2%	2%	2%	2%	1%	2%
Wales	–	–	2%	2%	2%	2%	1%	1%	2%	1%	1%
Scotland	–	1%	3%	4%	2%	1%	1%	2%	1%	2%	1%
Northern Ireland	1%	1%	3%	4%	2%	1%	2%	1%	1%	1%	2%
United Kingdom	–	1%	2%	2%	2%	2%	2%	2%	1%	1%	1%
Proportion with one or more lateral incisors instanding											
England	–	–	1%	3%	5%	6%	6%	6%	5%	5%	5%
Wales	–	–	3%	3%	4%	5%	7%	4%	6%	3%	7%
Scotland	–	–	1%	4%	4%	5%	6%	5%	4%	4%	3%
Northern Ireland	–	–	2%	3%	5%	4%	6%	5%	4%	6%	4%
United Kingdom	–	–	1%	4%	5%	6%	7%	6%	4%	5%	5%
Proportion with one or more incisors instanding											
England	–	1%	3%	4%	7%	7%	6%	6%	6%	5%	6%
Wales	–	–	5%	4%	5%	7%	7%	4%	6%	3%	7%
Scotland	–	1%	4%	7%	6%	5%	6%	5%	5%	6%	3%
Northern Ireland	1%	1%	5%	7%	6%	5%	7%	5%	4%	7%	5%
United Kingdom	–	1%	3%	4%	7%	7%	7%	6%	6%	5%	5%

For bases see Appendix A

Table 10.20   The proportion of children with one or more edge-to-edge permanent incisors by country

	Age (years)										
	5	6	7	8	9	10	11	12	13	14	15
Proportion with one or more edge-to-edge central incisors											
England	–	1%	2%	2%	1%	2%	2%	2%	2%	2%	4%
Wales	–	–	4%	2%	2%	1%	1%	3%	1%	2%	3%
Scotland	–	1%	1%	2%	2%	3%	2%	3%	2%	3%	2%
Northern Ireland	–	–	1%	2%	1%	1%	2%	1%	2%	3%	2%
United Kingdom	–	1%	2%	2%	2%	2%	2%	2%	2%	2%	4%
Proportion with one or more edge-to-edge lateral incisors											
England	–	–	1%	2%	4%	6%	4%	4%	6%	6%	8%
Wales	–	–	1%	1%	1%	3%	2%	3%	4%	3%	6%
Scotland	–	–	1%	3%	4%	5%	4%	4%	5%	4%	5%
Northern Ireland	–	–	2%	2%	5%	2%	4%	3%	5%	3%	6%
United Kingdom	–	–	1%	2%	4%	6%	4%	4%	6%	5%	8%
Proportion with one or more edge-to-edge incisors											
England	–	1%	3%	6%	5%	7%	5%	5%	7%	7%	11%
Wales	–	–	5%	4%	2%	4%	3%	6%	4%	4%	8%
Scotland	–	1%	2%	4%	5%	6%	5%	6%	5%	6%	7%
Northern Ireland	–	–	2%	3%	6%	3%	5%	5%	6%	6%	8%
United Kingdom	–	1%	3%	5%	5%	7%	5%	5%	7%	8%	9%

For bases see Appendix A

Table 10.21   The proportion of children with one or more rotated permanent incisors by country

	Age (years)										
	5	6	7	8	9	10	11	12	13	14	15
England	–	1%	6%	8%	7%	5%	4%	4%	4%	4%	5%
Wales	–	2%	10%	15%	14%	9%	11%	7%	9%	8%	8%
Scotland	–	1%	3%	4%	5%	3%	2%	3%	4%	3%	5%
Northern Ireland	–	1%	4%	10%	10%	16%	7%	13%	8%	9%	9%
United Kingdom	–	1%	6%	8%	8%	5%	4%	4%	4%	4%	5%

For bases see Appendix A

Table 10.22 The proportions of children with traumatic overbite

	Age (years)										
	5	6	7	8	9	10	11	12	13	14	15
England	–	–	1%	2%	2%	3%	1%	2%	2%	2%	1%
Wales	–	–	1%	–	2%	1%	1%	1%	1%	1%	1%
Scotland	–	–	1%	1%	1%	–	–	–	1%	1%	–
Northern Ireland	–	–	3%	3%	4%	2%	1%	3%	1%	3%	–
United Kingdom	–	–	1%	2%	2%	2%	1%	1%	2%	2%	1%

For bases see Appendix A

Table 10.23 The proportions of children with crowding

	Age (years)										
	5	6	7	8	9	10	11	12	13	14	15
England	1%	17%	54%	69%	71%	66%	67%	62%	63%	62%	66%
Wales	1%	20%	52%	69%	69%	72%	69%	65%	63%	58%	52%
Scotland	1%	13%	40%	58%	55%	63%	59%	60%	53%	56%	54%
Northern Ireland	2%	18%	51%	60%	65%	71%	58%	57%	51%	48%	51%
United Kingdom	1%	17%	53%	68%	69%	67%	66%	62%	62%	61%	64%

For bases see Appendix A

Table 10.24 Proportion of children who have some permanent teeth missing due to decay

	Age (years)										
	5	6	7	8	9	10	11	12	13	14	15
England	–	–	–	2%	3%	5%	8%	12%	14%	16%	21%
Wales	–	–	–	2%	4%	8%	13%	17%	24%	24%	34%
Scotland	–	–	1%	4%	9%	15%	18%	25%	31%	39%	44%
Northern Ireland	–	–	2%	7%	11%	15%	26%	31%	41%	40%	53%
United Kingdom	–	–	–	2%	4%	6%	10%	14%	16%	19%	24%

For bases see Appendix A

The removal of teeth to make extra room in the mouth is a way of alleviating crowding, but if teeth have been extracted for other reasons, for example because they were decayed, this will also make extra room in the jaw. Reference to Table 10.24 shows that a much higher proportion of children in Scotland and Northern Ireland had a permanent tooth missing due to decay. Among fourteen year olds, for example, 40% of the children from Northern Ireland and 39% of the children from Scotland had lost permanent teeth through dental decay compared with 24% from Wales and just 16% from England. Thus this greater loss of teeth due to decay among children in Scotland and Northern Ireland is likely to be related to the lower proportions of children with crowded teeth in those countries.

Generally, in the United Kingdom as a whole, the average number of teeth missing due to decay and the average number of teeth which had been orthodontically extracted were very similar (Table 10.25). Among fourteen year olds there was a slightly higher average number of teeth that had been orthodontically extracted than were missing due to decay.

Table 10.25 Average number of permanent teeth extracted for orthodontic reasons and average number missing due to decay

Age (years)	Average number of permanent teeth	
	Orthodontically extracted	Missing due to decay
5	–	–
6	–	–
7	–	–
8	–	–
9	–	0.1
10	–	0.1
11	0.2	0.2
12	0.4	0.3
13	0.5	0.4
14	0.7	0.4
15	0.7	0.6

10.6 Orthodontic treatment

During the dental examination the dentist recorded whether or not a child was wearing an orthodontic appliance and also asked the child whether they had ever had an appliance. This information can be combined with information that was collected concerning orthodontic extractions to give a fuller picture of a child's orthodontic treatment history. In the introduction to this chapter (Table 10.2) it was shown that the majority of children in the United Kingdom do not receive orthodontic treatment; by the age of fifteen one third of the children had received treatment of some kind. Table 10.26 shows how the provision of treatment varies between children in the constituent countries of the United Kingdom (for ease of presentation those children aged ten and under are omitted from the table as there was so little treatment experience in these age groups).

Table 10.26 Treatment history

Treatment history	Age (years)					
	10	11	12	13	14	15
	%	%	%	%	%	%
England						
Under treatment now	2	4	9	9	6	5
Had treatment						
Extractions only	1	4	5	7	9	13
Appliance only	3	3	2	4	4	6
Extractions and appliance	–	1	3	6	10	13
Never had treatment	94	88	81	74	71	63
Total	100	100	100	100	100	100
Wales						
Under treatment now	2	4	6	10	9	5
Had treatment						
Extractions only	1	4	6	8	9	10
Appliance only	2	5	2	4	3	4
Extractions and applicance	–	1	1	6	11	11
Never had treatment	95	86	85	72	68	70
Total	100	100	100	100	100	100
Scotland						
Under treatment now	–	3	4	6	6	2
Had treatment						
Extractions only	1	4	7	7	7	9
Appliance only	5	3	4	5	6	6
Extractions and appliance	1	1	4	7	7	11
Never had treatment	93	89	81	75	74	72
Total	100	100	100	100	100	100
Northern Ireland						
Under treatment now	1	2	5	7	8	6
Had treatment						
Extractions only	–	1	3	5	5	6
Appliance only	3	4	2	4	4	2
Extractions and appliance	–	1	1	3	5	6
Never had treatment	94	92	89	81	78	80
Total	100	100	100	100	100	100

For bases see Appendix A

Generally it can be seen that in the age groups twelve and over the highest proportion of children who had never had orthodontic treatment was found in Northern Ireland although there was no statistically significant difference in this proportion between the twelve year olds in Northern Ireland and the twelve year olds in Wales nor between the fourteen year olds in Northern Ireland and the fourteen years olds in Scotland. Looking at the proportions of children currently wearing an appliance it can be seen that there were no obvious differences over all ages between children in the constituent countries. However, among twelve year olds there was a significantly higher proportion of children currently wearing an appliance in England (9%) than in Scotland (4%) or Northern Ireland (5%), among fourteen year olds there was a significantly higher proportion in Wales (10%) than in England (6%) or Scotland (5%) and among fifteen year olds there were significantly higher proportions in England (5%) and Northern Ireland (6%) than in Scotland (2%).

It is of interest to note that there is no evidence of a substantially lower proportion of children in Northern Ireland than elsewhere currently wearing an appliance yet reference to the table shows that among the older children, proportionately fewer from Northern Ireland had worn an appliance in the past compared with children in the other countries. This suggests that appliance therapy is as common now in Northern Ireland as it is elsewhere but that it may only have become so in recent years.

For those orthodontic appliances that were being worn at the time of the dental examination, the dentist recorded whether they were of a fixed type or whether they were of a removable type. The vast majority were of the removable type with just 15% being of a fixed type.

10.7 Orthodontic treatment need

We have seen how much orthodontic treatment had been provided for children and in this section we look at the proportions of children who were, in the dentists' opinion, in need of orthodontic treatment.

For each child who had some permanent upper incisors present and who was not currently undergoing ortho-

dontic treatment, the dentist recorded whether, in his opinion, the child was in need of orthodontic treatment (or assessment for orthodontic treatment) and, if so, for what feature or features this was needed. This was a subjective judgement by the dentist and did not necessarily relate directly to the assessment the dentist had made about the occlusion of the teeth. For example, the dentist may have recorded a child as having crowded teeth, but not, in fact, have felt that the child needed treatment to correct this.

It can be seen from Table 10.27 that the highest proportion of children who, in the dentist's opinion, needed assessment for orthodontic treatment, were the eight and nine year olds and that these proportions decreased among the older children. (The proportions of children who needed orthodontic treatment were also lower in the age groups under eight but this was due to the fact that a much smaller proportion of these children were assessed for orthodontic need because a

large number had no permanent upper incisors present.) There are two likely reasons why orthodontic need decreases among the older children. First, as the jaw develops problems of oral alignment may be resolved naturally. Second, we have already seen that the proportions of children who had received orthodontic treatment were higher among the older children and therefore this past treatment will have been directed at some earlier need for treatment among the older children. We look in more detail at the relationship between past orthodontic treatment and current orthodontic need later in this section.

Looking at the variation in the proportions of children with an orthodontic need between the constituent countries of the United Kingdom, it can be seen that except among the oldest and youngest children there were signficantly higher proportions of children who were in need of orthodontic treatment in Wales than in any of the other countries. England, Scotland and

Table 10.27 The proportion of children with some orthodontic need

	Age (years)										
	5	6	7	8	9	10	11	12	13	14	15
England	1%	9%	39%	55%	56%	52%	46%	40%	34%	32%	31%
Wales	1%	18%	56%	69%	69%	65%	60%	50%	42%	38%	28%
Scotland	1%	8%	31%	47%	47%	47%	41%	39%	27%	28%	21%
Northern Ireland	1%	10%	35%	50%	50%	53%	39%	49%	37%	36%	35%
United Kingdom	1%	9%	39%	55%	56%	52%	46%	41%	34%	32%	30%

Table 10.28 The proportion of children with orthodontic need; what feature is in need of treatment

	Age (years)										
	5	6	7	8	9	10	11	12	13	14	15
	Proportion who need treatment for crowding										
England	1%	7%	32%	45%	47%	42%	38%	33%	28%	27%	26%
Wales	–	17%	49%	63%	61%	56%	52%	41%	36%	33%	32%
Scotland	1%	5%	24%	38%	39%	40%	35%	32%	22%	22%	17%
Northern Ireland	1%	8%	28%	39%	38%	39%	30%	39%	31%	27%	30%
United Kingdom	1%	7%	33%	46%	47%	43%	38%	33%	28%	27%	25%
	Proportion who need treatment for overjet										
England	–	2%	11%	17%	16%	15%	14%	13%	9%	8%	7%
Wales	1%	1%	8%	15%	18%	18%	14%	16%	8%	6%	5%
Scotland	–	2%	7%	11%	12%	10%	9%	7%	5%	7%	4%
Northern Ireland	–	–	7%	12%	11%	13%	7%	10%	4%	7%	5%
United Kingdom	–	2%	10%	16%	16%	15%	13%	12%	8%	8%	6%
	Proportion who need treatment for an instanding incisor										
England	–	1%	3%	4%	7%	7%	6%	5%	5%	3%	4%
Wales	–	1%	5%	4%	5%	5%	6%	2%	4%	3%	5%
Scotland	–	1%	4%	7%	3%	4%	5%	4%	3%	4%	3%
Northern Ireland	–	–	5%	7%	4%	4%	6%	4%	3%	4%	4%
United Kingdom	–	1%	4%	4%	6%	7%	6%	5%	4%	3%	4%
	Proportion who need treatment for a rotated incisor										
England	–	–	3%	4%	5%	4%	4%	2%	2%	3%	3%
Wales	–	2%	7%	10%	10%	6%	8%	3%	5%	5%	4%
Scotland	–	1%	3%	5%	4%	3%	3%	3%	3%	3%	2%
Northern Ireland	–	–	1%	3%	4%	6%	2%	6%	3%	4%	2%
United Kingdom	–	1%	3%	5%	6%	4%	4%	2%	3%	3%	3%
	Proportion who need treatment for gingival trauma										
England	–	1%	1%	1%	1%	2%	1%	1%	1%	1%	1%
Wales	–	–	1%	–	1%	1%	1%	1%	1%	1%	–
Scotland	–	–	1%	1%	1%	1%	1%	1%	1%	1%	1%
Northern Ireland	–	–	1%	1%	2%	1%	1%	1%	1%	1%	1%
United Kingdom	–	1%	1%	1%	1%	2%	1%	1%	1%	1%	1%

For bases see Appendix A

Northern Ireland had similar proportions of children who needed orthodontic treatment, although among the eight and nine year olds there were higher proportions of children in England than in Scotland who needed treatment and among the older children there was a higher proportion in Northern Ireland than in Scotland who needed orthodontic treatment.

Table 10.28 shows the dentists' assessments of the orthodontic conditions that, in their opinion, required treatment. Generally, for each of the conditions assessed, the need for treatment was found to be greatest among the eight to ten year olds. The most common treatment needed was that to correct crowded teeth; among the eight and nine year olds in the United Kingdom almost half the children seen were in need of this type of treatment. Much smaller proportions of children were recorded as needing treatment for other conditions with for example, 16% of nine year olds needing treatment to correct their overjet, 6% needing treatment because of an instanding incisor, 6% needing treatment because of a rotated incisor and 1% needing treatment because of gingival trauma.

It was shown earlier in this section that the highest proportions of children found to be in need of orthodontic treatment were those from Wales and it can be seen from Table 10.28 that this is mainly due to the much higher levels of children who were in need of treatment for crowding (although there were slightly higher proportions of children in Wales who needed treatment for a rotated incisor). Looking back to Table 10.22 it can be seen that there were not significantly higher proportions of children in Wales recorded as having crowding. We looked to see whether there was a higher proportion of children in Wales with crowding in the anterior segments, which might have been considered more serious but this was not the case. It was left to the dentists' subjective view as to whether a child was in need of orthodontic treatment and so we looked at the calibration trials that took place before the survey to see whether the Welsh dentists had been more likely than others to assess the mouth as crowded,

but again this was not the case. One can only assume that among the children in Wales there was a particular type of crowding that was more likely to be recorded by the dentist as needing treatment to correct it.

It has been shown that there was a relatively high proportion of children in the middle age range who were, in the dentists' opinion, in need of orthodontic treatment and that this proportion was smaller among the older children. As was stated earlier this may be due to the older children having received treatment to correct orthodontic anomalies. Thus it is of interest to relate a child's treatment history to the assessment of orthodontic need. In Table 10.3 in the introduction to this chapter, the relationship between overall treatment need and past treatment was presented. Here we look at the two features most commonly found to be in need of treatment, overjet and crowding, to see how their presence is related to a child's treatment history. It should be noted that we do not have information as to the reason for past treatment, only about whether or not a child had received any treatment.

Table 10.29 shows the proportions of children aged ten and over who in the dentists' opinion needed treatment to correct overjet according to whether or not they had ever had any orthodontic treatment. It can be seen that the proportion of children who had never had orthodontic treatment but who needed treatment to correct overjet decreased with age from 15% of ten year olds to 4% of fifteen year olds. It can also be seen that the proportion of children who had had orthodontic treatment and who had no treatment need increased with age. These results imply that the need for treatment to correct increased overjet is generally being met. This result is shown more clearly in terms of crowded teeth (Table 10.30). The proportions of children who needed treatment for crowded teeth and who had not had any past treatment decreased with age from 42% of the ten year olds to 18% of the fifteen year olds, while the proportion of children who were not in need of treatment and who had had past orthodontic treatment increased from 3% of the ten year olds to 20% of the fifteen year olds.

Table 10.29 Need for orthodontic treatment to correct an increased overjet

Need for orthodontic treatment	Age (years)					
	10	11	12	13	14	15
	%	%	%	%	%	%
Had no orthodontic need	43	46	45	47	47	45
Had treatment in the past and:						
Needs treatment for overjet	–	–	1	1	1	2
Needs treatment for other reason	2	4	3	6	6	8
No longer needs treatment	3	4	6	11	15	20
Had not had treatment in past and:						
Needs treatment for overjet	15	12	11	7	7	4
Needs treatment for other reason	35	31	25	20	18	16
Under treatment now	1	3	9	8	6	5
Total	100	100	100	100	100	100

For bases see Appendix A

Table 10.30 Need for orthodontic treatment to correct crowding

Need for orthodontic treatment	Age (years)					
	10	11	12	13	14	15
	%	%	%	%	%	%
Had no orthodontic need	43	46	45	47	47	45
Has had treatment in the past and:						
Needs treatment for crowding	1	3	3	5	6	7
Needs treatment for other reason	1	1	1	2	1	3
No longer needs treatment	3	4	6	11	15	20
Has not had treatment in past and:						
Needs treatment for crowding	42	35	30	24	21	18
Needs treatment for other reason	9	7	7	3	4	3
Under treatment now	1	3	9	8	6	5
Total	100	100	100	100	100	100

For bases see Appendix A

10.8 Summary

The survey dental examination collected three kinds of information about the orthodontic situation of children. It provided an estimate of the prevalence of various orthodontic anomalies as defined in the examination criteria. It provided some information about orthodontic treatment experience in terms of whether children had previously had orthodontic extractions or had worn orthodontic appliances or were currently under treatment for orthodontic reasons. It also provided an estimate by the survey dental examiner as to whether in his/her opinion the child required orthodontic treatment or an assessment for orthodontic treatment. The orthodontic conditions for which measurements were made were overjet, rotation of incisors, instanding or edge-to-edge incisors, increased overbite causing trauma and crowding, but these measures were not in themselves indications of treatment need.

Nearly three quarters of children who were examined with respect to the orthodontic criteria had one or more of the following conditions, an overjet of 5 mm or more, an incisor that was rotated, instanding or in an edge-to-edge relationship, traumatic injury due to an increased overbite or crowding of the teeth. For children aged twelve, 20% had received some orthodontic treatment, a proportion that rose with age until at age fifteen a third of children had received some orthodontic treatment. Among children aged eight, nine and ten over half were said by the survey dental examiner to have not yet had orthodontic treatment but to be in need of it. This proportion declined among the older children but it was still estimated that a quarter of fourteen year olds and a fifth of fifteen year olds had not had orthodontic treatment and needed it.

It was clear from the findings that it was crowding of the teeth that was by far the most common developmental anomaly found among the children. Among children aged 11 – 14 there were lower proportions with crowded teeth in Northern Ireland than in England or Wales. Earlier chapters have shown that the proportion of children with permanent teeth extracted due to decay was higher in Northern Ireland and Scotland than elsewhere.

When the dental examiners made their assessments as to which children required treatment for crowding this was by no means all those who had been recorded as having crowding. From the age of eight about two thirds of children were said to have some crowding but just under half of the youngest and a quarter of the oldest were said to need treatment for it.

11 Orthodontic assessments 1973 and 1983

11.1 Introduction
The section of the examination that covered the orthodontic assessment in 1983 was not identical to that used in 1973. Certain measurements were excluded from the 1983 examination and others were made using different criteria. In addition, the orthodontic assessments were made in 1983 only when a child had at least one permanent upper incisor present whereas in 1973 all children had been examined for the orthodontic assessment. In this chapter comparisons made between the two surveys are restricted to measures which were directly comparable, and to children aged eight and over, to ensure that only valid comparisons are made.

11.2 Incisor problems
Table 11.1 shows the proportions of children with at least one incisor that was either instanding or in an edge-to-edge relationship, and it can be seen that there was very little difference between the prevalence of these conditions in 1973 and in 1983. (There is an apparent increase in the proportion of fifteen year olds with incisor problems but it should be noted that, as explained in the report on the 1973 survey, the sample of fifteen year olds in that study was not truly representative as it contained only those fifteen year olds who had stayed on at school after the statutory leaving age. One should therefore be cautious about making comparisons over the ten years for this age group.)

Table 11.2 shows that there was no difference between 1973 and 1983 in the proportions of children with a zero or negative overjet measurement. Neither was there any difference between the proportions with a large measurement of overjet.

11.3 Crowding
Crowding was assessed using similar criteria in both 1973 and 1983. In 1983 information was also collected about orthodontic extractions so that results could be presented showing past treatment to alleviate crowding. This analysis was not carried out in 1973 but a comparison can be made between crowding as measured using the same criteria in 1973 and 1983. In England and Wales, the proportion of children with crowding increased substantially between 1973 and 1983 (Table 11.3). For example, the proportion of thirteen year olds with some crowding increased from 52% in 1973 to 65% in 1983 and the proportion of fourteen year olds with some crowding increased from 50% in 1973 to 63% in 1983.

Table 11.1 The proportion of children with an instanding or edge-to-edge incisor: England and Wales, 1973 and 1983

Age (years)	1973	1983
8	12%	9%
9	11%	10%
10	11%	12%
11	10%	10%
12	9%	10%
13	9%	11%
14	10%	10%
15	9%	13%

For bases see Appendix A

Table 11.2 Proportion of children with extremes of overjet (upper central incisor): England and Wales, 1973 and 1983

Age (years)	Proportion with overjet measurement of:					
	Zero or negative		5–6 mm		7mm or more	
	1973	1983	1973	1983	1973	1983
8	4%	3%	11%	16%	7%	8%
9	2%	3%	12%	13%	6%	9%
10	3%	3%	12%	13%	5%	9%
11	3%	3%	15%	14%	6%	7%
12	3%	3%	11%	13%	7%	8%
13	3%	4%	11%	11%	3%	7%
14	4%	4%	11%	10%	4%	5%
15	3%	5%	11%	12%	3%	4%

For bases see Appendix A

Table 11.3 The proportion of children with crowding: England and Wales, 1973 and 1983

Age (years)	1973	1983
8	65%	70%
9	63%	73%
10	62%	69%
11	58%	69%
12	55%	65%
13	52%	65%
14	50%	63%
15	53%	66%

For bases see Appendix A

Table 11.4 Proportion of children who have had orthodontic extractions compared with the proportion who have had decay extractions: England and Wales, 1973 and 1983

Age (years)	Proportion who have had:			
	Orthodontic extractions		Decay extractions	
	1973	1983	1973	1983
8	–	–	4%	2%
9	1%	–	8%	3%
10	2%	2%	13%	5%
11	7%	7%	18%	9%
12	13%	15%	23%	13%
13	17%	19%	28%	15%
14	22%	24%	31%	17%
15	21%	29%	33%	22%

For bases see Appendix A

It can be seen from Table 11.4 that the proportion of children who had had teeth extracted for decay reasons decreased sharply between the two surveys. For example, among fourteen year olds the proportion who had some permanent teeth extracted for decay reasons decreased from 31% in 1973 to 17% in 1983. The proportion of children who had had teeth extracted for orthodontic reasons, however, did not vary between 1973 and 1983. Thus it can be seen that in 1973 there was generally less potential for overcrowding than in 1983. In 1973 more teeth on average had been lost for decay reasons than in 1983 thus creating space in the mouth.

11.4 Orthodontic treatment and need

In the previous section we saw that there had been no increase in the proportion of children who had received orthodontic treatment in the form of orthodontic extractions. Table 11.5 shows the proportions of children who had orthodontic treatment in the form of an appliance. During the dental examination in both 1973 and 1983 the dentist asked the children whether they had ever worn a brace and, also, recorded whether each child was wearing a brace at the time of the examination. Table 11.5 shows that, as in the case of orthodontic extractions, there was no significant difference between the proportion of children who were receiving or had received orthodontic appliance therapy in 1983 and the proportion in 1973.

In addition to there having been no change in the level of provision of orthodontic treatment between 1973 and 1983, there was also no statistically significant difference between the proportions of children said, by the dentist, to be in need of orthodontic treatment (Table 11.6).

It was seen earlier that there had been a significant rise in the proportion of children with crowded teeth, yet there was no rise in the proportion of children in need of orthodontic treatment. However, as was noted in the previous chapter, the presence of crowding, as with the other orthodontic assessments was recorded by the dentist regardless of whether or not the dentist felt it needed treatment to correct it. Thus the proportion of children recorded as having crowding was much higher than the proportion recorded as needing treatment for crowding.

Table 11.5 Proportion of children who had had appliance therapy: England and Wales, 1973 and 1983

Age (years)	Proportion who:			
	Had a brace at the examination		Had had a brace	
	1973	1983	1973	1983
8	–	–	1%	1%
9	–	–	1%	1%
10	1%	1%	2%	4%
11	3%	3%	4%	5%
12	5%	7%	7%	7%
13	4%	6%	10%	12%
14	2%	4%	13%	16%
15	1%	3%	16%	20%

For bases see Appendix A

Table 11.6 Proportion of children in need of orthodontic treatment: England and Wales, in 1973 and 1983

Age (years)	Proportion in need of orthodontic treatment	
	1973	1983
8	57%	56%
9	55%	57%
10	50%	53%
11	46%	47%
12	37%	41%
13	30%	34%
14	28%	32%
15	27%	31%

For bases see Appendix A

Due to different methods of collecting the dental data we cannot compare the reasons the dentist thought that the child needed treatment for 1973 and 1983. So though we can see that there had been no rise in the orthodontic need of children as assessed by the dental examiners we do not know whether this assessment was based on similar or different aspects of treatment need.

11.5 Summary

Although there were certain differences between the orthodontic examination in the 1973 and the 1983 survey certain aspects of these examinations were comparable. There was in fact no difference between children in 1973 and 1983 in the proportion who had orthodontic anomalies connected with the incisors. The proportion of children recorded as having some crowding or potential crowding was higher in 1983 than it had been ten years earlier. The number of permanent teeth extracted due to decay had, on the other hand been higher in 1973 than ten years later. Despite this difference in the recorded level of crowding as defined by the survey examination criteria, the proportion of children said to be in need of orthodontic treatment in 1983 was not higher than it had been in 1973.

12 Parental attitude to orthodontic treatment

12.1 Introduction

In the previous chapters results have been presented showing the provision of orthodontic treatment and the assessment of orthodontic need. Although a dentist may suggest that a child undergoes orthodontic treatment, the perception by the parent that the child has an orthodontic problem will play a part in whether or not the child receives treatment. In this chapter, therefore, we look at the parent's attitudes towards the occlusion of their children's teeth and see how this is related to the dental assessment of orthodontic need. Information was collected from the parents of the children aged five, eight, twelve and fifteen but because orthodontic assessments were not made for the youngest children we confine the analyses in this chapter to the older children.

12.2 Crowding

In the previous chapters we saw that the orthodontic condition that was most prevalent and the one that the dentist recorded most often as in need of treatment was overcrowded teeth. In the survey, parents were asked: "*At this stage of growing up are any of your child's teeth crooked at all, or not?*" and Table 12.1 shows how the answers they gave related to the dentist's assessment of whether or not the child needed treatment for crowding.

It can be seen that of those children who the dentist said did not need treatment, approximately three quarters of the parents said that they did not think their children's teeth were crooked. Among those children who the dentist recorded as being in need of treatment for crowding, a higher proportion of parents agreed with the dentist that the child's teeth were crooked. For example, among twelve year olds who needed treatment for crowding, 48% of the parents agreed that the teeth were crooked. This proportion was slightly lower with regard to the eight year olds (41%) and the fifteen year olds (39%). It may be that at eight years old, parents are less worried about the look of their children's teeth because they think that any problems will sort themselves out naturally at a later date, while by the time the age of fifteen has been reached, the parents may have become used to the appearance of their children's teeth and less likely to remark on crowded teeth. Among eight year olds and twelve year olds there were no large differences between boys and girls in the parent's perception of crooked teeth. However, among fifteen year olds whom the dentist said needed treatment for crowding, a higher proportion of parents said that girls teeth were crooked than said the same for boys.

Table 12.1 Parental attitude to crowding by dental assessment of whether treatment needed to correct crowding and sex of child

Sex of child and parental attitude	Age (years) and dental assessment					
	8		12		15	
	No treatment need	Treatment need	No treatment need	Treatment need	No treatment need	Treatment need
Male	%	%	%	%	%	%
Teeth not crooked	76	59	77	50	81	62
Teeth crooked	23	39	21	47	16	34
Don't know	1	2	2	3	3	4
Total	100	100	100	100	100	100
Base	*274*	*201*	*366*	*204*	*402*	*144*
Female						
Teeth not crooked	75	55	75	49	80	55
Teeth crooked	24	43	23	48	19	44
Don't know	1	2	2	3	1	1
Total	100	100	100	100	100	100
Base	*220*	*218*	*370*	*167*	*412*	*129*
Both sexes						
Teeth not crooked	75	57	76	49	81	59
Teeth crooked	24	41	22	48	17	39
Don't know	1	2	2	3	2	2
Total	100	100	100	100	100	100
Base	*493*	*420*	*736*	*371*	*815*	*275*

Table 12.2 Parental attitude to crowding by dental assessment of need for treatment for crowding by whether or not had orthodontic treatment

Parental attitude	Age (years)							
	12				15			
	Treatment in past†		No treatment in past		Treatment in past†		No treatment in past	
	No treatment need	Treatment need	No treatment need	Treatment need	No treatment need	Treatment need	No treatment need	Treatment need
	%	%	%	%	%	%	%	%
Teeth not crooked	53	40	84	50	65	57	90	59
Teeth crooked	46	57	14	47	32	39	9	39
Don't know	1	3	2	3	3	4	1	2
Total	100	100	100	100	100	100	100	100
Base	179	37	556	334	355	83	516	190

† It is not recorded for what reasons the past treatment was supplied

A curious result is shown in Table 12.2 regarding parents attitudes to crowding according to whether or not a child had, in the past, received orthodontic treatment. (Because so few eight year olds had received treatment only the twelve and fifteen year olds are shown.) Parents whose children had received orthodontic treatment in the past and who were said by the dentist not to currently need treatment for crowding, were much more likely to say that their child's teeth were crooked than were the parents of children who had not had orthodontic treatment but had no need for such treatment. For example among twelve year olds who, according to the dentist, did not need treatment for crowding, 46% of the parents of children who had received orthodontic treatment said they thought their children's teeth were crooked compared with 14% for children who had not had treatment in the past. Although parents were specifically asked about the current situation, it may be that parents of children who had had treatment in the past were conscious of the fact that their children's teeth had once been crooked and thus a proportion of them may have erroneously recorded that their children's teeth were currently crooked.

12.3 Protruding teeth

In addition to asking parents whether they thought that their children's teeth were crooked, we also asked whether they thought their child's teeth were 'protruding or sticking out'. In Table 12.3 we look at how the parents' view was related to the assessment of whether or not a child was said to need treatment to correct the overjet. For children with a reported need for such treatment, a relatively high proportion of parents said that they did not think their children's teeth protruded. The figure was 68% in the case of eight year olds, 58% for twelve year olds and 76% for fifteen year olds. A higher proportion of parents of girls needing treatment thought that their children's teeth did protrude compared with parents of boys. For example among fifteen year olds with a treatment need, 28% of parents of girls thought that their child's teeth protruded compared with 20% of parents of boys.

Table 12.3 Parental attitude to protruding teeth by dental assessment of treatment need to correct overjet, by sex of child

Sex of child and parental attitude	Age (years) and dental assessment					
	8		12		15	
	No treatment need	Treatment need	No treatment need	Treatment need	No treatment need	Treatment need
Male						
	%	%	%	%	%	%
Teeth do not protrude	87	70	83	64	89	79
Teeth protrude	10	28	15	32	8	20
Don't know	3	2	2	4	2	1
Total	100	100	100	100	100	100
Base	398	77	491	79	510	37
Female						
Teeth do not protrude	85	66	81	51	89	72
Teeth protrude	12	32	18	44	10	28
Don't know	2	2	2	4	1	–
Total	100	100	100	100	100	100
Base	365	73	478	59	509	33
Both sexes						
Teeth do not protrude	86	68	82	58	89	76
Teeth protrude	11	30	16	37	9	24
Don't know	3	2	2	4	2	–
Total	100	100	100	100	100	100
Base	763	150	969	138	1,019	70

Among the parents of children aged twelve and fifteen who had no need for orthodontic treatment to correct overjet, a higher proportion of those whose children had received such treatment in the past than of those who had not, said that their children's teeth protruded (Table 12.4). The differences between the two groups were not as large however as those seen (above) when we looked at whether or not parents thought their children's teeth were crooked by whether or not they had previously had treatment.

12.4 Orthodontic treatment need

Regardless of whether or not the parents had said that they thought their children's teeth were protruding or crooked, all parents whose children were not currently receiving orthodontic treatment were asked: *"At the moment do you think your children's teeth are alright as they are or would you prefer them to be straightened?"*. Table 12.5 shows how the parent answers are related to whether or not the dentist recorded the child to be in need of any orthodontic treatment or not.

Generally, a high proportion of parents were satisfied with their children's teeth and only a minority wanted them to be straightened. Among children whom the dentist recorded as being in need or orthodontic treatment, the highest proportion of children whose parents would have liked their children's teeth to be straightened was found among the twelve year olds, particularly among the girls. Generally, though, there is little apparent demand from the parents for orthodontic treatment.

Table 12.4 **Parental attitude to protruding teeth by dental assessment of need for treatment to correct overjet measure by whether or not had orthodontic treatment**

Parental attitude	Age (years)							
	12				15			
	Treatment in past†		No treatment in past		Treatment in past†		No treatment in past	
	No treatment need	Treatment need	No treatment need	Treatment need	No treatment need	Treatment need	No treatment need	Treatment need
	%	%	%	%	%	%	%	%
Teeth do not protrude	70	*	86	60	86	*	91	78
Teeth protrude	29	*	12	36	12	*	8	21
Don't know	1	*	2	5	2	*	2	1
Total	100	100	100	100	100	100	100	100
Base	*182*	*12*	*764*	*126*	*350*	*21*	*658*	*48*

* Percentages not given for bases of less than 30
† It is not recorded for what reasons the past treatment was supplied

Table 12.5 **Parental attitude to children's teeth by dental assessment of orthodontic treatment need, by sex of child**

Sex of child and parental attitudes	Age (years) and dental assessment					
	8		12		15	
	No treatment need	Treatment need	No treatment need	Treatment need	No treatment need	Treatment need
Male						
	%	%	%	%	%	%
Teeth alright as they are	90	82	92	75	93	81
Prefer them to be straightened	8	17	6	23	3	15
Don't know	2	1	2	2	4	4
Total	100	100	100	100	100	100
Base	*201*	*234*	*259*	*205*	*338*	*163*
Female						
Teeth alright as they are	85	77	91	64	94	83
Prefer them to be straightened	12	21	6	32	4	15
Don't know	3	2	2	4	2	2
Total	100	100	100	100	100	100
Base	*165*	*235*	*261*	*165*	*343*	*142*
Both sexes						
Teeth alright as they are	88	80	91	70	93	82
Prefer them to be straightened	10	19	6	27	4	15
Don't know	3	1	2	3	3	3
Total	100	100	100	100	100	100
Base	*366*	*469*	*520*	*370*	*681*	*305*

Table 12.6 Parental attitude to children's teeth by dental assessment of orthodontic treatment need by whether or not had orthodontic treatment

Parental attitude	Age (years)							
	12				15			
	Treatment in past		No treatment in past		Treatment in past		No treatment in past	
	No treatment need	Treatment need	No treatment need	Treatment need	No treatment need	Treatment need	No treatment need	Treatment need
	%	%	%	%	%	%	%	%
Teeth alright as they are	90	69	92	76	94	83	93	87
Prefer them to be straightened	5	31	7	26	5	15	3	15
Don't know	5	–	2	4	2	2	3	4
Total	100	100	100	100	100	100	100	100
Base	*60*	*31*	*460*	*339*	*211*	*95*	*471*	*210*

It is interesting to see from Table 12.6 that, unlike the case of crowded or protruding teeth, the fact that a child has had orthodontic treatment in the past is not seen to affect the attitude of the parents as to whether or not they would like their children's teeth to be straightened.

12.5 Summary

Parents were asked some questions about what they thought about the appearance of their child's teeth, especially whether they thought the teeth were crooked or protruding, and they were asked whether they would like their child to have his/her teeth straightened. Among children whom the dentist assessed as not needing any orthodontic treatment for crowding about four out of five parents said their child's teeth were not crooked. However among those for whom the dentist said there was an orthodontic treatment need for reasons of crowding fewer than half the parents said the child's teeth were crooked. The results thus show that crowding that was of dental significance to the examiner was not recognised as being a problem by over half of the parents.

13 Accidental damage to the teeth

13.1 Introduction

During the dental examination the dentist assessed each permanent incisor for evidence of accidental damage. For each incisor with evidence of such damage the dentist recorded the type of damage sustained and any treatment which the child had received for that damage. In this chapter we look at the prevalence of traumatic injury and treatment provided in the United Kingdom in 1983.

Also presented in this chapter is a comparison of the levels of trauma found in England and Wales in 1983 with results from the 1973 survey. In 1983, the assessment of accidental damage had been made only on permanent incisors whereas in 1973 the assessment was carried out on both dentitions. Comparisons can therefore only be made among the older children, for whom data is available from both surveys.

13.2 The prevalence of traumatic injury

Table 13.1 shows the proportions of children in the constituent countries of the United Kingdom who had sustained some type of accidental damage to their permanent incisors. (The results are presented only for those children aged eight and over because among these children virtually all of the permanent incisors were present.) Generally, it can be seen that in the United Kingdom as a whole, the proportion of children with some accidental damage increased with age, up to

the age of thirteen and that among the thirteen to fifteen year olds the proportion with some injury remained constant at about one quarter. It is perhaps not surprising to note that traumatic injury was more common among boys than among girls, due most probably to the rougher nature of boys activities. In fact, among the older boys, one third were found to have some kind of accidental damage to their permanent incisors compared with just one fifth of the older girls.

13.3 Accidental damage and treatment

Nationally, there were no large differences in the proportion of children with some traumatic injury to their incisors, although among the fifteen year olds there was a slightly higher proportion of children in Wales with such damage than in the other countries.

The type of accidental damage that was recorded ranged from an enamel fracture or discolouration to the actual loss of a tooth. The type of treatment recorded for traumatic injury ranged from minor restorations to the replacement of the missing tooth by a denture. The results are shown in Table 13.2, for all eight incisors together and for the upper central incisors separately, the latter being most at risk for traumatic damage. The results are presented in terms of how many incisors there were in each condition per thousand incisors seen by the dentist.

Table 13.1 The prevalence of accidental damage among children aged eight and over by sex

Age (years)	England	Wales	Scotland	Northern Ireland	United Kingdom
Males					
8	13%	9%	9%	6%	12%
9	15%	18%	14%	11%	15%
10	18%	18%	17%	14%	18%
11	24%	28%	20%	25%	24%
12	29%	31%	29%	22%	29%
13	29%	33%	27%	27%	29%
14	33%	35%	31%	27%	33%
15	34%	35%	28%	30%	33%
Females					
8	7%	6%	8%	5%	7%
9	9%	10%	6%	7%	9%
10	14%	16%	15%	11%	14%
11	18%	16%	10%	15%	17%
12	16%	12%	15%	13%	16%
13	23%	24%	18%	14%	22%
14	17%	16%	18%	16%	17%
15	19%	27%	21%	19%	19%
Both sexes					
8	10%	8%	9%	5%	10%
9	12%	14%	10%	9%	12%
10	16%	17%	16%	13%	16%
11	21%	22%	15%	21%	21%
12	23%	22%	23%	18%	23%
13	26%	28%	22%	20%	26%
14	26%	27%	25%	21%	25%
15	26%	30%	25%	24%	26%

For bases see Appendix A

Table 13.2 Type of accidental damage sustained per 1,000 incisors for children aged eight and over

Type of damage	Age (years)							
	8	9	10	11	12	13	14	15
All incisors								
Discolouration	0.2	0.6	0.5	0.3	1.8	1.7	1.7	3.7
Fracture (enamel)	9.2	12.4	15.8	23.9	24.5	30.2	26.4	28.9
Fracture (enamel & dentine)	4.7	5.1	7.5	7.0	8.9	7.8	10.7	8.7
Fracture (involving pulp)	0.3	0.1	0.4	0.2	0.5	1.3	0.9	1.4
Missing due to trauma	0.3	0.6	0.6	0.6	0.9	0.5	0.3	1.6
Acid etch restoration	1.8	3.9	3.3	4.4	4.2	6.0	6.0	5.1
Permanent crown	–	0.1	0.4	1.1	1.4	1.8	1.7	3.6
Other restoration	0.1	0.1	0.6	0.4	0.3	0.6	0.7	0.8
Denture due to trauma	0.3	–	–	0.6	0.4	0.5	0.3	1.5
Upper central incisors								
Discolouration	0.6	2.6	2.2	1.0	5.8	4.8	6.3	9.9
Fracture (enamel)	29.4	32.4	43.0	66.4	72.7	81.4	75.6	81.3
Fracture (enamel & dentine)	15.8	15.5	22.2	21.4	25.2	19.7	31.9	24.6
Fracture (involving pulp)	1.2	0.5	1.0	0.6	1.8	3.6	3.0	3.8
Missing due to trauma	1.1	1.2	1.7	2.3	2.6	1.9	1.1	4.3
Acid etch restoration	7.2	13.7	12.8	15.7	13.7	21.5	20.0	16.6
Permanent crown	–	0.5	1.4	3.8	5.5	5.8	5.2	11.3
Other restoration	0.2	0.3	2.4	1.4	0.9	2.0	2.3	2.2
Denture due to trauma	1.0	–	0.1	2.3	1.8	2.4	1.5	4.3

The prevalence of each type of damage was higher for each year of age, except in the case of a fracture involving both the enamel and dentine, where the prevalence was lower among the fifteen year olds, compared with the fourteen year olds. For example, among fourteen year olds there were 31.9 upper central incisors per thousand upper central incisors with a fracture involving both enamel and dentine compared with 24.6 per thousand among the fifteen year olds. Similarly, the presence of each type of treatment for traumatic injury was higher with each increase in age, except in the case of acid etch restorations which were lower among the oldest children (for example, there were 5.1 acid etch restorations per thousand incisors among fifteen year olds compared with 6.0 per thousand among thirteen and fourteen year olds).

Of the different types of damage sustained, the type most commonly recorded was a fracture involving the enamel only. Among fifteen year olds, for example, 28.9 incisors per thousand were recorded as having this damage, while 81.3 upper central incisors per thousand upper central incisors were recorded in this way. As expected, compared with all incisors, the upper central incisors had suffered more damage in each of the recorded categories.

Of each of the different types of treatment recorded, the most frequent type found was acid etch restorations, particularly on the upper central incisors. For example, among thirteen year olds, per thousand upper central incisors, there were 21.5 acid etch restorations compared with 5.8 permanent crowns, 2.4 dentures and 2.0 other types of restoration.

It is obvious from Table 13.2 that the prevalence of damage to the incisors, exceeds by far the prevalence of treatment. This is shown more clearly in Table 13.3 where the children who had some accidental damage are analysed by whether or not any treatment was recorded for that damage. It can be seen that in the vast majority of cases, trauma had not been treated. Among twelve year olds for example, only 10% of incisors with traumatic injury had been treated. There was little systematic variation with age or, indeed, sex although the highest proportions of treated traumatic injury occurred among the nine year olds and among the fifteen year olds. (In these age groups the proportions of damaged incisors which had been treated were 18% and 16% respectively.)

Table 13.3 Proportions of accidental damage that have and have not been treated for children aged eight and over by sex

	Age (years)							
	8	9	10	11	12	13	14	15
Males	%	%	%	%	%	%	%	%
Treated trauma	11	18	13	13	11	9	14	15
Untreated trauma	89	82	87	87	89	91	86	85
Total	100	100	100	100	100	100	100	100
Females								
Treated trauma	16	17	12	12	7	15	12	19
Untreated trauma	84	83	88	88	93	85	88	81
Total	100	100	100	100	100	100	100	100
Both sexes								
Treated trauma	12	18	13	13	10	11	13	16
Untreated trauma	88	82	87	87	90	89	87	84
Total	100	100	100	100	100	100	100	100

For bases see Appendix A

Table 13.4 Accidental damage for children with different measures of overjet

	Age (years)							
	8	9	10	11	12	13	14	15
	%	%	%	%	%	%	%	%
	Children with an overjet of less than 5mm							
Some trauma	9	10	12	16	21	22	21	22
No trauma	91	90	88	84	79	78	79	78
Total	100	100	100	100	100	100	100	100
Base	*687*	*796*	*887*	*930*	*909*	*989*	*1,061*	*948*
	Children with an overjet of 5mm or more							
Some trauma	13	21	28	33	27	36	38	39
No trauma	87	79	72	67	73	64	62	61
Total	100	100	100	100	100	100	100	100
Base	*232*	*233*	*253*	*247*	*245*	*215*	*187*	*185*

13.4 Traumatic injury and overjet

In this section, we look at the relationship between protruding teeth and traumatic injury of the incisors, in that one might expect a higher level of traumatic injury among children whose teeth protruded.

Table 13.4 shows the presence of traumatic injury for children with an overjet of less than 5mm and for children with an overjet of 5mm or more (which has been taken as an indication of protruding teeth). The table shows clearly that a higher proportion of children with an increased overjet have traumatic injury to their incisors compared with those with an overjet of less than 5mm. For example, among thirteen year olds, 22% of children with an overjet of less than 5mm have sustained traumatic injury to their incisors compared with 36% of those with an overjet of 5mm or more.

It is of interest to see whether the prevalence of trauma increases among children with very large overjets. However, as we saw from Chapter 10, very few children have such large overjets. In Table 13.5, therefore, we have combined age groups to show the prevalence of trauma among children with an overjet of 9mm or more. It can be seen from the table that there is strong evidence to suggest that the larger the overjet the more likely children are to damage their incisors. Among children aged twelve and over, nearly one half of children with an overjet of 9mm or more had accidental damage to their incisors.

Table 13.5 Accidental damage for children with large overjets

	Age (years)			
	8–9	10–11	12–13	14–15
	%	%	%	%
	Children with an overjet of less than 9mm			
Some trauma	11	17	23	24
No trauma	89	83	77	77
Total	100	100	100	100
Base	*1,888*	*2,248*	*2,287*	*2,320*
	Children with an overjet of 9mm or more			
Some trauma	7	34	45	44
No trauma	93	66	55	56
Total	100	100	100	100
Base	*61*	*70*	*71*	*49*

13.5 Traumatic injury 1973 and 1983

The 1973 dental examination included an assessment of traumatic damage on both the permanent and deciduous dentition. Thus if we wish to make comparisons between accidental damage in England and Wales in 1973 and 1983, we must confine ourselves to the older children for whom all permanent incisors can be assumed to be present. In addition to excluding the deciduous teeth from the assessment in 1983, some changes were made to the recording of the different categories for treatment of trauma and thus, we confine the analysis of change only to the assessment of the type of traumatic injury sustained.

Additionally, initial analysis showed that there was a very large reported increase in the number of incisors with fractured enamel, that is, the least serious traumatic injury. It would seem unlikely that there has in fact been such a large increase in this type of injury over this period. It would seem more likely that the difference between the two sets of results represents a change in diagnostic assessment among the dental team. It may be that for some reason over the ten years between 1973 and 1983 the dental profession has become more aware of this type of damage. We concluded that with respect to the measurement of fractured enamel we were not comparing like with like between the two surveys and therefore confined the analyses to those types of traumatic injury where we believe we have comparability between 1973 and 1983.

Table 13.6 shows the rate of accidental damage to the incisors per thousand incisors in 1973 and 1983 for all eight incisors and for the upper central incisors.

It can be seen that both in the case of all incisors and the upper central incisors, for children aged thirteen and over there has been a rise in the number of teeth discoloured due to trauma. For example, among fourteen year olds in 1973 there were 2.2 per thousand upper central incisors discoloured due to trauma compared with 5.4 per thousand in 1983.

Looking at all eight incisors, there was a slight rise in the rate of fractures that involved both enamel and dentine in all age groups except the twelve year olds. In

Table 13.6 Traumatic injury in England and Wales, 1973 and 1983

Type of damage	Age (years)											
	10		11		12		13		14		15	
	1973	1983	1973	1983	1973	1983	1973	1983	1973	1983	1973	1983
Rate of damage (per thousand) incisors												
Discolouration	0.5	0.5	0.5	0.2	2.4	1.5	0.5	1.4	0.7	1.5	0.9	3.7
Fracture (enamel and dentine)	6.5	7.8	7.6	8.7	8.6	8.7	5.7	7.8	9.2	10.7	7.5	8.1
Fracture (involving pulp)	0.6	0.4	1.0	0.3	1.0	0.3	1.2	1.3	2.6	0.7	0.9	1.4
Missing due to trauma	–	0.5	0.9	0.7	1.3	0.7	1.6	0.5	1.1	0.2	1.1	1.5
Rate of damage (per thousand) upper central incisors												
Discolouration	1.8	2.1	2.0	0.8	6.3	4.8	1.1	4.4	2.2	5.4	2.9	10.0
Fracture (enamel and dentine)	20.6	23.2	21.8	22.2	23.0	25.1	20.2	19.2	21.7	33.0	21.6	23.3
Fracture (involving pulp)	1.8	1.0	4.1	0.5	2.1	1.3	4.4	3.9	3.8	2.2	3.6	4.1
Missing due to trauma	–	1.5	3.5	2.5	4.7	1.9	5.5	2.1	3.8	1.0	2.9	4.2

the case of the upper central incisors there was a large rise in the rate of fractures involving enamel and dentine among the fourteen year olds (from 21.7 per thousand in 1973 to 33.0 per thousand in 1983).

The rate per thousand incisors of all eight incisors which had a fracture which involved the pulp was lower among all but the thirteen and fifteen year olds in 1983 than in 1973 while the rate of fractures involving pulp among the upper central incisors was less in all but the oldest age group.

There were fewer incisors missing due to trauma in the age range eleven to fourteen in 1983 than in 1973. For example, among twelve year olds, 4.7 per thousand upper central incisors were missing due to trauma in 1973 compared with 1.9 per thousand in 1983.

Thus, generally, it would seem that in 1983 as compared with 1973 there was a slightly higher level of the less severe forms of accidental damage, such as discolouration, but a slightly lower level of the more severe forms of accidental damage such as the loss of a tooth through trauma.

13.6 Parental knowledge of accidental damage

The previous sections presented information about the proportions of children who had sustained traumatic injury to a permanent incisor as measured at the dental examination. This section presents information taken from the questionnaire relating to damage to the incisors. The dental assessment covered only permanent incisors that had evidence of traumatic injury, so in order to get an impression of total experience of such damage we asked parents whether their child had *"ever had a fall or some other accident that damaged any of his/her teeth?"*, and if they said they had, they were asked whether it was the deciduous or permanent dentition that was involved.

It is immediately obvious from the answers given (Table 13.7) and from reference back to Table 13.1 that parents are not as aware of accidental damage to teeth as the dental examiners. The proportion of children who were recorded in the examination as having damaged permanent incisors was much higher than the proportion of children whose parents said they had damaged their permanent incisors. For example,

Table 13.7 Proportion of children who have, according to their parents damaged their incisors

	Age (years)			
	5	8	12	15
	Proportion with traumatic injury			
Deciduous incisors	14%	12%	7%	6%
Permanent incisors	–	6%	13%	16%
Any damage	14%	18%	19%	22%

For bases see Appendix A

among 15 year olds the dentist recorded 26% with traumatic injury while the parents of just 16% said they had damaged a permanent incisor.

Even allowing for the fact that the parents may confuse permanent and deciduous teeth, the proportion of children in the older age groups who were classified by the dentist as having traumatic injury to a permanent incisor was higher than the proportion of children who were said by their parents to have had any damage at all to their incisors.

Table 13.8 shows whether or not the parents knew of accidental injury to the permanent incisors for all children for whom the dentist recorded accidental damage. (The five year olds are omitted as the dental examiners only recorded damage evident on the permanent incisors.) About a half of the parents whose children had sustained traumatic injury to their permanent incisors, reported that their children had damaged teeth. (This was about the same level of awareness that was reported in England and Wales in 1973.)

Table 13.8 Proportion of parents who said child had damaged a permanent tooth among children whom the dentist had classified as having traumatised incisors

Whether parents said child had damaged permanent teeth	Age (years)		
	8	12	15
	%	%	%
Some damage	43	47	46
No damage	57	53	53
Don't know	–	–	1
Total	100	100	100
Base	*89*	*247*	*288*

Table 13.9 Proportion of parents who said child had damaged a permanent tooth among children whom the dentist classified as having a traumatised incisor (apart from solely fractured enamel).

Whether parents said child had damaged permanent teeth	Age (years)		
	8	12	15
	%	%	%
Some damage	82	78	73
No damage	18	22	26
Don't know	–	–	1
Total	100	100	100
Base	*34*	*94*	*115*

It was shown earlier that the majority of damage recorded was of a fairly mild type, namely a fracture of the enamel and we felt that it was maybe not surprising that parents were unaware of this type of damage. Table 13.9 shows whether or not the parents said that their child had damaged a permanent incisor for those children who the dentist recorded as having a traumatised incisor, excluding those where the only damage was a fracture of the enamel. It can be seen that, in this case, a much higher proportion of the parents were aware that the child had damaged a tooth. For twelve year olds, for example, of those that had some damage to their incisors apart from just a fracture of the enamel, 78% of the parents said that their child had damaged a permanent incisor.

13.7 Summary

In 1983 accidental damage was only recorded with respect to the permanent dentition. Although the criteria were intended to be comparable there was in 1983 a large increase in the number of teeth recorded as having fractured enamel compared with the situation in 1973. This would seem to have arisen from an increase in awareness of this condition within the profession rather than any change in criteria.

There was no marked variation in the level of traumatised incisors in the different countries of the United Kingdom. Boys were more likely to have suffered such damage than girls, and by and large the prevalence of trauma was higher at each succeeding year of age, the teeth having been at risk for longer. By the age of fifteen 81 per 1,000 central incisors were recorded as having fractured enamel, 4 per 1,000 were missing due to trauma, 2 per 1,000 had been replaced by a denture, 11 per 1,000 had a permanent crown and 17 per 1,000 had an acid etch restoration. Children with large overjets were more likely than those with small overjets to have damaged incisors. In the period 1973 to 1983, ignoring the increased level of fractured enamel that was recorded, there was a slight rise in the less serious kinds of damage and a slight decrease in the more serious kinds of injury.

Parents had a reasonable awareness of the more serious kinds of damage. If children who only had teeth that were damaged to the extent of having fractured enamel were excluded then three quarters of the parents of children with more serious trauma were able to tell us that their child had had some kind of accident.

14 Children's dental health in Wales

14.1 Introduction

When the 1973 survey of children's dental health was carried out in England and Wales, the sample of children in Wales was enhanced so that separate results could be presented for that country. We have already presented information collected from children in Wales in 1983 in previous chapters of the report, but in this chapter we provide a direct comparison for a selection of the findings from the 1983 survey together with the results from the 1973 survey for Wales.

14.2 Known decay experience of the deciduous teeth

In this section we look at the known decay experience of the deciduous dentition for children in Wales in 1973 and 1983. Table 14.1 shows the proportion of children with some known decay experience in the deciduous teeth, that is, the proportion of children with some decayed deciduous teeth and/or some filled deciduous teeth. In the ages five to nine there was a decrease in the proportion of children with known decay experience in the deciduous dentition between 1973 and 1983. This decrease was largest among the youngest children. Among six year olds, for example, the proportion with some known deciduous decay experience decreased from 83% in 1973 to 68% in 1983. Among children over the age of nine, that is among those who had already lost many of their deciduous teeth, the proportion of children with some known decay experience increased between 1973 and 1983.

Table 14.1   Proportion of children with known decay experience in their deciduous teeth: Wales, 1973 and 1983

Age (years)	1973	1983
5	78%	66%
6	83%	68%
7	86%	69%
8	88%	80%
9	84%	78%
10	57%	65%
11	38%	42%
12	20%	25%
13	6%	10%
14	2%	2%
15	1%	1%

For bases see Appendix A

From Tables 14.2 and 14.3 it can be seen that this increase in decay experience was due to an increase among children of all ages in Wales in the proportion who had a filled deciduous tooth (Table 14.3). Among the five year olds the proportion with some filled deciduous teeth increased from 22% in 1973 to 35% in 1983 while among the ten and eleven year olds the proportions with some filled deciduous teeth doubled. This increase in restorative treatment helped children retain for longer deciduous teeth that had become decayed.

Table 14.2   Proportion of children with some active decay in the deciduous teeth: Wales, 1973 and 1983

Age (year)	1973	1983
5	71%	48%
6	74%	54%
7	79%	53%
8	79%	62%
9	74%	58%
10	50%	45%
11	32%	29%
12	14%	17%
13	5%	7%
14	1%	1%
15	1%	1%

For bases see Appendix A

Table 14.3   Proportion of children with some filled (otherwise sound) deciduous teeth: Wales, 1973 and 1983

Age (years)	1973	1983
5	22%	35%
6	30%	38%
7	33%	40%
8	38%	47%
9	34%	48%
10	19%	43%
11	12%	26%
12	8%	11%
13	1%	5%
14	1%	2%
15	1%	–

For bases see Appendix A

The proportion of children in Wales with some actively decayed deciduous teeth decreased between 1973 and 1983 among children aged five to ten (Table 14.2), while among the older children the proportions were similar in 1973 and 1983. Among the younger children there were some particularly large decreases in the proportion with some active decay. Among five year olds, for example, 71% of children in Wales in 1973 had some actively decayed deciduous teeth while in 1983 the figure was 48%.

Taking these three results together, that is the proportion of children with some decayed deciduous teeth, the proportion with some filled deciduous teeth and the proportion with some filled and/or some decayed deciduous teeth, it would seem that in 1983 in Wales, deciduous teeth were being filled which in 1973 would have been left with active decay or maybe even lost due to decay. This would explain both the increase in the proportion of children with some filled teeth and the decrease in the proportion of children with some decayed teeth. However, because the proportion of children with some teeth that were decayed and/or some teeth which were filled decreased in the younger age groups, it can also be concluded that there has been a reduction in dental disease between the two surveys.

In terms of the average number of deciduous teeth with known decay experience, that is either decayed or filled, it can be seen that, up to the age of ten, there was a large decrease between the two surveys (Table 14.4). For example, among six year olds in Wales the average number of decayed or filled deciduous teeth decreased from 4.2 in 1973 to 2.7 in 1983. This decrease was due to the decrease in the average number of teeth that were actively decayed (among six year olds, for example, from 3.4 teeth to 1.7 teeth). There was an increase in the average number of deciduous filled teeth, among eight year olds, for example, the average was 0.9 teeth in 1973 and 1.3 in 1983.

Table 14.5 Proportion of children with known decay experience in the permanent teeth: Wales, 1973 and 1983

Age (years)	1973	1983
5	3%	1%
6	24%	6%
7	43%	16%
8	67%	40%
9	75%	53%
10	87%	65%
11	91%	78%
12	98%	83%
13	97%	86%
14	98%	94%
15	99%	94%

For bases see Appendix A

Table 14.4 Average number of deciduous teeth with known decay experience: Wales, 1973 and 1983

Age (years)	Average number of deciduous teeth					
	Decayed		Filled		Decayed and/or filled	
	1973	1983	1973	1983	1973	1983
5	3.5	1.8	0.5	0.8	4.0	2.6
6	3.4	1.7	0.8	1.0	4.2	2.7
7	3.2	1.4	0.8	1.0	4.0	2.4
8	2.6	1.5	0.9	1.3	3.5	2.8
9	2.3	1.4	0.8	1.2	3.2	2.7
10	1.3	0.9	0.4	1.0	1.7	1.9
11	0.6	0.5	0.2	0.5	0.8	1.0
12	0.3	0.3	0.1	0.2	0.4	0.5
13	0.1	0.1	0.0	0.1	0.1	0.2
14	–	–	–	–	–	–
15	–	–	–	–	–	–

For bases see Appendix A

14.3 Known decay experience of permanent teeth

The decrease in decay experience, observed in the deciduous dentition in children in Wales between 1973 and 1983, was also apparent in the permanent dentition. Table 14.5 shows the proportions of children with some permanent teeth which were decayed, filled or missing due to decay. The decreases in the proportions were particularly marked among the younger children. Among seven year olds, for example, the proportion of children with some known decay experience in their permanent dentition decreased from 43% in 1973 to 16% in 1983.

The proportion of children in Wales with some actively decayed permanent teeth also decreased between the two surveys (Table 14.6). Among fourteen year olds in 1973, 71% had aome permanent teeth which were actively decayed. In 1983 this figure was 42%. Similarly the proportion of children with some teeth which had been extracted because of decay decreased. Among the fourteen year olds this figure decreased from one half to one quarter (Table 14.7).

In the previous section we saw that the proportion of children in Wales with some filled deciduous teeth had increased over the ten years. However, this was not true for filled permanent teeth (Table 14.8). In fact, there was very little change between the two surveys in the proportion of children in Wales with some filled permanent teeth.

Table 14.6 Proportion of children with some active decay in the permanent teeth: Wales, 1973 and 1983

Age (years)	1973	1983
5	3%	1%
6	19%	5%
7	33%	8%
8	50%	17%
9	49%	21%
10	59%	21%
11	63%	37%
12	68%	33%
13	70%	40%
14	71%	42%
15	71%	46%

For bases see Appendix A

Table 14.7 Proportion of children with some teeth missing due to decay: Wales, 1973 and 1983

Age (years)	1973	1983
5	–	–
6	–	–
7	2%	–
8	6%	2%
9	14%	4%
10	22%	8%
11	32%	13%
12	38%	17%
13	45%	24%
14	50%	24%
15	50%	34%

For bases see Appendix A

Table 14.8 Proportion of children with some filled teeth in the permanent dentition: Wales, 1973 and 1983

Age (years)	1973	1983
5	–	1%
6	7%	2%
7	14%	9%
8	28%	29%
9	41%	40%
10	52%	53%
11	55%	58%
12	71%	72%
13	71%	74%
14	70%	83%
15	88%	87%

For bases see Appendix A

Table 14.9 Average numberof permanent teeth with known decay experience: Wales, 1973 and 1983

Age (years)	Average number of permanent teeth							
	Decayed		Missing		Filled		Decayed, missing and/or filled	
	1973	1983	1973	1983	1973	1983	1973	1983
5	–	–	–	–	–	–	–	–
6	0.4	0.1	–	–	0.1	0.0	0.5	0.1
7	0.7	0.1	–	–	0.3	0.2	1.0	0.3
8	1.0	0.3	0.1	0.0	0.6	0.6	1.7	0.9
9	1.2	0.4	0.3	0.1	1.0	0.8	2.4	1.3
10	1.4	0.4	0.5	0.2	1.4	1.2	3.3	1.8
11	1.9	0.8	0.6	0.3	1.5	1.6	4.1	2.6
12	2.0	0.7	1.0	0.3	2.5	2.3	5.5	3.3
13	2.6	0.9	1.1	0.5	3.1	3.0	6.9	4.5
14	2.9	1.1	1.4	0.5	4.3	4.0	8.6	5.6
15	2.6	1.2	1.5	0.8	5.9	4.8	10.1	6.7

For bases see Appendix A

Table 14.10 Dental attendance patterns: Wales, 1973 and 1983

Attendance pattern	Age (years)							
	5		8		12		14	15
	1973	1983	1973	1983	1973	1983	1973	1983
	%	%	%	%	%	%	%	%
Regular attenders	34	44	40	55	46	59	43	57
Occasional attenders	5	18	9	12	8	15	17	19
Only when having trouble	61	37	51	32	46	24	40	23
All attenders	100	100	100	100	100	100	100	100

For bases see Appendix A

From Table 14.9 it can be seen that, in Wales, the average number of permanent teeth with known decay experience decreased between 1973 and 1983. In each of the age groups from nine upwards, at least one fewer tooth on average had decay experience in 1983 than had been the case in 1973. Among fourteen year olds there was a reduction in the average of three teeth, from 8.6 in 1973 to 5.6 in 1983. Large reductions were also seen, between 1973 and 1983, in the average number of permanent teeth that were actively decayed and the average number of teeth missing due to decay. There were no large changes in the average number of filled permanent teeth. There was a slight indication of a decrease in this average among the older children but, as has been noted before, the sample of fifteen year olds in 1973 was not truly representative as a section of them had already left school and were thus not examined. One should be wary therefore of drawing conclusions from comparisons of the oldest age group.

14.4 Changes in attendance patterns

It has been shown that the state of children's dental health in Wales as for the whole of England and Wales improved substantially between 1973 and 1983. In this section we look briefly at an indicator of dental attitudes to see whether there were similar improvements. The regularity and purpose for which the parent says that the child visits the dentist is an indicator of the child's dental background and the importance that is placed on dental health in the family. In both 1973 and 1983, we grouped children with like dental attendance patterns using information given by the parents about the length of time since the last visit to the dentist and the reason for the last visit. Those who had been to the dentist in the previous six months for a check-up were classified as regular attenders, those whose last visit was for a check-up but was longer ago than six months were classed as occasional attenders, and those whose last visit was because of dental problems or because the school dentist had advised that the child visit the dentist, were classed as those who attend the dentist only when having trouble with their teeth. (This latter category also included those children who had never visited the dentist.)

Table 14.10 shows the reported attendance patterns for children in Wales in 1973 and 1983. In each of the age groups the proportion of regular attenders increased by at least ten percentage points. Similarly the proportion who attend the dentist only when having trouble with their teeth declined. For example among twelve year olds in 1973, 46% were said to be regular attenders and 46% were said to attend only when having trouble with their teeth. In 1983, 59% were said to be regular attenders and just 24% were said to attend only when having trouble with their teeth.

Thus we can see that the improvement in dental health in Wales as measured by the dental examination has been accompanied by an increase in dental awareness as indicated by the increase in the proportions of children who are said to attend a dentist for a regular check-up.

14.5 Summary

Separate estimates for the dental health of children in Wales were made in both 1973 and 1983. The situation for Wales in 1983 has been given throughout the report as part of the comparison between the countries of the United Kingdom. In this chapter direct comparisons are made for Wales over the ten year period from 1973 to 1983.

With respect to the deciduous dentition there was a reduction between 1973 and 1983 in known decay experience amongst the younger children in Wales (aged 5–9) and an increase among the older children. The increase among the older children was due to an increase in the number of filled deciduous teeth which had therefore been retained longer and thus signified an improvement in dental care.

For the permanent dentition there was also a reduction in known decay experience. The reduction was particularly marked in the permanent dentition of some of the youngest children.

There were fewer children with active decay in their permanent teeth and fewer that had already lost permanent teeth due to decay, and about the same proportion with filled permanent teeth. The results thus show a considerable change in the amount of disease in the permanent dentition comparing 1973 with 1983.

Over this period there had also been a change, for the better, in the proportion of children who are said to go to the dentist for a regular check-up rather than only when they have trouble with their teeth. Reductions in the level of disease and an improved awareness of dental care among children in Wales makes prospects for dental health encouraging for the next decade.

Appendix A Base numbers

Total children examined 1983

Age (years)	England	Wales	Scotland	Northern Ireland
5	671	190	319	198
6	717	211	357	202
7	772	225	357	201
8	811	213	412	202
9	891	262	401	225
10	983	249	416	224
11	989	272	479	233
12	971	258	525	239
13	991	281	507	276
14	1,042	264	588	227
15	967	279	486	217

Weighted bases 1983

Age (years)	England and Wales	United Kingdom
5	719	804
6	770	863
7	829	921
8	865	968
9	957	1,061
10	1,046	1,152
11	1,058	1,177
12	1,036	1,165
13	1,062	1,192
14	1,109	1,248
15	1,038	1,156

Regions of England and Wales 1983

Age (years)	The North	Midlands and East Anglia	Wales and the South West	London and the South East
5	221	151	102	245
6	232	156	105	277
7	245	199	126	259
8	260	218	113	274
9	323	219	140	275
10	328	259	134	325
11	327	239	147	345
12	319	233	143	341
13	308	231	157	366
14	356	258	151	344
15	334	233	151	320

Total response from parents 1983

Age (years)	England	Wales	England and Wales	Scotland	Northern Ireland	United Kingdom
5	630	180	675	303	170	756
8	766	207	818	387	175	914
12	923	251	986	493	226	1,109
15	915	260	980	444	190	1,089
Social class of household						
I, II, III N						
5	277	66	294	104	62	321
8	323	71	341	128	62	373
12	346	92	369	153	74	407
15	356	95	380	153	55	416
III M						
5	219	67	236	127	67	268
8	258	73	276	167	58	315
12	331	94	355	204	86	404
15	314	98	339	164	64	378
IV, V						
5	87	36	96	49	23	108
8	130	47	142	68	33	159
12	155	54	169	94	40	191
15	154	50	167	91	45	189

Attendance pattern 1983

Age (years)	England	Wales	England and Wales	Scotland	Northern Ireland	United Kingdom
Regular check-up						
5	358	79	377	126	44	407
8	480	114	508	202	87	558
12	590	149	627	292	89	694
15	543	149	580	226	71	632
Occasional check-up						
5	109	32	117	33	30	127
8	90	24	96	33	25	105
12	102	38	112	57	45	128
15	168	50	180	76	40	200
Only with trouble						
5	153	66	170	133	94	207
8	185	66	202	146	57	236
12	209	61	224	139	86	261
15	184	59	199	135	76	234

Base numbers for 1973 survey

Age (years)	Children examined		Parents interviewed	
	England and Wales	Wales alone	England and Wales	Wales alone
5	952	172	922	168
6	1,080	184		
7	1,137	191		
8	1,091	183	532	90
9	1,129	195		
10	1,092	182		
11	986	176		
12	956	175	451	87
13	915	185		
14	923	177	886	174
15	696	120		

England and Wales 1973	Age (years)			
	5	8	12	14
Social class				
I, II, III N	283	177	165	284
III M	441	227	174	396
IV, V	158	108	92	176
Attendance pattern				
Regular check-up	357	268	234	421
Occasional check-up	76	54	64	169
Only with trouble	485	208	148	293

Appendix B The training of the dentists
(by the Departments of Dental Health at the Universities of Birmingham and Newcastle)

Introduction
The planning of this study took place when feeling was growing that national information was essential because there were indications from local sources that the dental health of school children was changing. The organisers were also aware of the high costs of previous surveys and knew that financial restraint would be necessary. For these reasons it was necessary to ensure that any changes in the design and conduct of the study would not affect the validity of comparisons made with findings of the former investigation and would allow the cost to be kept to within a reasonable budget.

Changes in design and method
One of the major sources of expenditure in the previous study had been the employment by OPCS of field staff. Their role had been to interview parents of the selected sample, to organise the dental fieldwork and to act as recorders and organisers during the period of the dental examinations. OPCS had evidence indicating that the interview information could be collected as reliably by postal questionnaire. As the dental examiners were to be recruited from the community dental services it was suggested that they could be accompanied by their own dental surgery assistants acting as recorders. Regional organisers recruited to assist with the training exercise would be chosen to liaise with the OPCS organisers during the fieldwork.

One beneficial aspect of having previously conducted two national dental surveys was that there existed a number of examiners who had been trained for previous studies and who were still available for participation in this one. Costs of training are particularly prohibitive since examiners from all parts of the UK need to travel to and be accommodated in one location for a fixed period of time. Although it was not feasible to reduce the travelling costs it was felt that by using experienced examiners the period of time necessary for their training could be reduced.

Previous dental surveys had incorporated a pilot study and a post calibration survey and consideration was given to omitting either or both of these exercises. It was decided that, with the proposed tailoring of the training exercise, and the differing fieldwork conditions, a pilot study was essential and should remain.

The post calibration exercises, in which all the examiners had been recalled to the training location after the completion of the data collection had resulted in no significant drift of examiner standardisation (1973 and 1978 studies). As many of them would be the same it was agreed that this exercise no longer justified the expense and therefore was not undertaken.

Establishing the criteria
Two potentially conflicting factors had to be considered in setting the criteria. The 1983 survey had to be a realistic up to date estimate of dental health but also permit comparisons with the 1973 study.

Meetings took place between the teams from the Dental Schools and the OPCS organisers during the summer of 1982 to determine the diagnostic and examination criteria. It was felt to be essential that the diagnostic criteria for caries remain identical to that used in 1983. The basic criteria for assessing oral hygiene and gum conditions should also remain the same but the WHO index would be introduced for older children.

The orthodontic assessment, although changed quite considerably on the data collection sheet to produce a more logical sequence of recording, was designed in such a way that comparisons could be made with the 1973 data. Examination for fissure sealants was introduced. As very few dentures were recorded in 1973 this section was removed and the section devoted to traumatised incisors was amended to record the presence of acid etch restorations and dentures placed due to traumatic injury.

Pre-pilot study
The pre-pilot study took place in the Children's Department of Newcastle Dental Hospital. Members of the organising teams acted as examiners and recorders to test the diagnostic criteria and the data collection document.

One aspect which caused concern to the organisers was the use of the WHO periodontal probe. Although the probe was found to be satisfactory, there were anticipated problems concerning adequate sterilising facilities. In the field the problem was resolved by supplying limited numbers of replaceable probe points to each examiner thus ensuring that each point was only used once before resterilisation. For this reason, this aspect of the periodontal examination was limited to the fifteen year old children.

Pilot study

In the adult study of 1978 the examiners who undertook the pilot study helped in the main training programme by acting as tutors. They were each responsible for a small group of examiners and guided them through the training exercise. As this link between examiners and organisers had proved to be successful it was decided to employ a similar system for the present study. They would also be able to play a valuable role as regional organisers during the field work, ensuring a link between the organisers and the dental team during the stage of the survey when the dental teams would be scattered throughout the UK.

Eight experienced epidemiologists were chosen as tutors, five from England and one each from Wales, Scotland and Northern Ireland. Although there was a meeting with them to discuss the mechanics of the pilot study and their co-ordinating role during the main study, no time was set aside during the pilot study to discuss the diagnostic and examination criteria. Instead copies of the criteria and an example of the charting procedure were sent to the pilot examiners prior to the training programme for study by them and their recorders alike.

The pilot study training exercise took place during the Autumn of 1982 at schools and a hotel in the Newcastle Upon Tyne area. Four different age groups of children were examined. The older children came from two secondary schools in Newcastle but because of the water fluoridation in that city it was felt that the younger children should come from outside the area. Accordingly two primary schools in Morpeth and Blyth were selected. Following the training exercise the examiners undertook a calibration exercise and examined a sample of children in their localities. After carrying out the pilot study the examiners reported back to the organisers matters arising during the exercise.

Main training courses

The training courses took place over two consecutive weeks for a period of two and half days each. With one half day being devoted to the calibration exercise two days remained for the training period. Copies of the diagnostic criteria, tape recorded examples of an examination and data collection documents were packaged with other instructions and information and sent to the examiners and the recorders prior to the course. They were requested to attain a working knowledge of the criteria and charting procedure by the time of their arrival in Newcastle. Other than an introductory meeting to clarify possible misunderstandings in the package, the training was undertaken by examining children in the schools used for the pilot study.

On the first day the dentists worked in pairs acting as either examiner or recorder for one half session and swapping roles for the second half of each session. Five year olds were examined in the mornings and eight year olds in the afternoons. This enabled the dentist to become familiar with both the criteria and coding systems and the role of the examiner and recorder. Any differences between examiners at this stage were monitored by the organisers and relayed back to the teams via the tutors.

On the second day the examiners were joined by their recorders and introduced to the administrative procedure of the fieldwork. The other half of the day was spent examining twelve and fifteen year olds. A calibration exercise took place on the third morning.

The Calibration study

On the final day of the training course a calibration exercise took place. This involved groups of dentists, with their dental nurses, examining groups of children in a situation similar to that they would find when they carried out the main fieldwork. No attempt was made to check the consistency of the dentists at the time of the calibration study but the results were analysed after the calibration so that a check could be made on the reliability of the different measures.

Two schools in the Newcastle area which had been used during the training courses kindly allowed us to visit them for a further morning session to carry out the calibration exercises. In each of the training weeks, two groups of dentists visited each school and each dentist carried out ten examinations. It was hoped that at each school, each of the dental teams that visited would be able to examine the same ten children and this was the case in one of the schools. However in the other school, certain children were not available at all the sessions and substitutions had to be made. We therefore carried out analyses on five groups; four small groups of dentists who saw four different groups of ten children and one large group of dentists who examined another group of ten children.

The results of such studies can be analysed in various ways and various different statistics can be produced to show the variation between dentists in their measurements. For the purpose of this report we present the results analysed in the way that has been employed on previous surveys so that readers may make comparisons if they wish.

Tables B1 and B2 show the variation within each of the groups of dentists on certain selected measurements. The less variability there is between dentists (and hence the more reliable a measure may be said to be) the smaller the coefficient of variation.

It can be seen, from Table B1, that in terms of measuring the health of the teeth, the measurements of the number of filled (otherwise sound) teeth, and the number of decayed, missing or filled teeth showed little variability; the value of the coefficient of variation in each of the groups was 0.1 or less.

The measurement of the number of actively decayed teeth showed a slightly higher degree of variation with coefficients of variation which ranged in value from 0.25 among Group B to 0.56 among Group E.

Table B1 Calibration results: caries and periodontal disease

	Groups of dentists				
	A	B	C	D	E
Number of dentists	10	7	9	10	37
Number of subjects	10	10	10	10	10
Actively decayed teeth					
Mean per dentists	5.7	6.3	7.7	6.9	9.1
Standard deviation	2.2	1.6	2.8	2.0	5.1
Coefficient of variation*	0.38	0.25	0.36	0.29	0.56
Filled otherwise sound teeth					
Mean per dentist	16.5	17.9	12.3	12.9	25.8
Standard deviation	1.0	0.5	1.2	0.9	1.7
Coefficient of variation*	0.06	0.02	0.09	0.07	0.07
Decayed, missing and filled teeth					
Mean per dentist	22.2	24.9	20.1	20.0	38.0
Standard deviation	1.6	2.2	1.8	1.6	4.0
Coefficient of variation*	0.07	0.09	0.09	0.08	0.10
Inflammation†					
Mean per dentist	2.6	14.1	2.9	14.7	12.2
Standard deviation	2.5	7.8	2.3	5.4	5.7
Coefficient of variation*	0.98	0.55	0.79	0.37	0.47
Debris†					
Mean per dentist	1.2	9.4	2.8	12.8	9.3
Standard deviation	1.7	6.3	2.9	8.3	5.5
Coefficient of variation*	1.42	0.67	1.03	0.65	0.59
Calculus†					
Mean per dentist	1.6	3.6	3.0	3.0	4.5
Standard deviation	0.7	2.6	1.6	1.3	2.7
Coefficient of variation*	0.41	0.75	0.54	0.45	0.60

* Coefficient of variation = $\dfrac{Standard\ deviation}{mean}$

† Number of segments with

Table B2 Calibration results: orthodontic assessments

	Groups of dentists				
	A	B	C	D	E
Number of dentists	10	7	9	10	37
Number of subjects	10	10	10	10	10
Size of overjet					
Mean per dentist (mm)	28.8	28.1	34.2	34.8	24.5
Standard deviation	3.0	2.7	3.5	3.4	7.8
Coefficient of variation*	0.10	0.10	0.10	0.10	0.30
Number of rotated incisors					
Mean per dentist	0.1	2.4	0.8	1.2	1.1
Standard deviation	0.3	2.1	0.4	0.7	0.6
Coefficient of variation*	3.00	0.88	0.53	0.62	0.55
Crowding					
Mean per dentist	13.3	14.7	11.7	15.3	12.4
Standard deviation	3.0	2.3	1.9	2.8	3.7
Coefficient of variation*	0.23	0.16	0.16	0.18	0.30
Number in need of treatment					
Mean per dentist	4.2	4.6	5.7	6.9	3.4
Standard deviation	1.5	1.4	0.8	1.8	1.4
Coefficient of variation*	0.35	0.31	0.14	0.25	0.41

* Coefficient of variation = $\dfrac{Standard\ deviation}{Mean}$

† Number of segments with

The variation in the assessment of the health of the gums was greater and, in the majority of cases, the coefficient of variation on each of the three measures inflammation, debris and calculus was larger than 0.5 with the assessment of the presence of debris showing a particularly high level of variability.

Table B2 shows the variability in the measurements of the orthodontic features. There was low variability on the measurement of overjet and relatively low levels of variability on the assessment of the number of segments with crowding and the assessment of whether or not a child was in need of orthodontic treatment.

There were very few children in the calibration study who had a rotated incisor and the assessment of this orthodontic feature gave rise to a high level of variability.

There were too few children included in the study with either instanding or edge-to-edge incisors or traumatic overbite to enable results to be presented for the variability of these measures.

Acknowledgements
We wish to acknowledge the Universities of Birmingham and Newcastle Upon Tyne for allowing us to take part in this study and the Newcastle Dental School and Hospital for the use of their facilities during the pre-pilot study.

We would like to thank Mr C L Carmichael, District Dental Officer, of Newcastle Health Authority and Mr A D French, District Dental Officer of Northumberland Health Authority for arranging the use of the schools in their respective districts. We are indebted to the headteachers, staff and children of the following schools; Horton Grange County First School, Blyth, Abbey Fields County First School, Morpeth, Heaton Manor Comprehensive School and Kenton Comprehensive School, Newcastle Upon Tyne. Without the enthusiastic participation of the children, the administrative assistance of the staff and the use of the school premises the training programme could not have succeeded.

Finally we wish to express our gratitude to all the dentists and nurses who travelled to Newcastle in winter conditions to undertake the intensive training course. The names of the examiners are listed in Appendix D.

Appendix C Materials sent to the dental team

Contents of packets for examiners/recorders

1 Details of necessary preparatory work.
2 The examination criteria.
3 The examination chart.
4 Examples of completed examination charts.
5 Description of charting procedures.
6 A miniature examination chart (for easy reference).
7 The programme for the training course.
8 A list of examiners and recorders.
9 A list of regional organisers names and addresses.
10 The grouping of examiners for the training course and the timetable for the groups.
11 A list of the equipment required.
12 Administrative details for the training course.
13 A claim form.

Main training

Equipment

Please bring with you the following items:
1 2 Towels.
2 A minimum of 4 mouth mirrors New No. 4 plain.
3 2 containers to hold mirrors and probes in antiseptic.
4 1 hand sponge.
5 1 polythene bag at least 1 ft square.
6 Clinical coat.
7 Angle-poise or similar lamp, with a 13 amp plug and a 60 watt single coil pearl bulb. (The examiners travelling from Northern Ireland do not have to bring this item.)
8 Pencils, rubbers, pencil sharpener.
9 A box of tissues or wipes.

We will provide:

1 Antiseptic during the training.
2 Caries probe.
3 Periodontal probe.
4 Orthodontic measure.
5 Extension leads for use at schools visited during training.

Please have the following items at your home before travelling to Newcastle so that they are ready for use on the Monday after your return.

1 A bottle of antiseptic.
2 An extension lead for your lamp with a plug or adaptor so that it will fit any socket.
3 An angle-poise lamp as described above. (Examiners travelling from Northern Ireland only.)

Preparatory work
On receipt of this package please will you undertake the following:

ON YOUR OWN

1 Check the contents of this package against the list of contents. Any omissions to be notified on the form in main packet received by examiner.
2 Make yourself familiar with the administrative details of the training course. In particular, identify your reference number. This number is important for identifying which group you are in during the course and, also, must be entered on all documents used during the examinations for the survey.
3 Read and become familiar with the examination criteria and the examination chart.
4 Listen to BOTH sides of the cassette tape, which was included in the main package. The examples of completed charts which you have are of the examinations on the tape. Compare one with the other.

WITH YOUR EXAMINER/RECORDER

1 Go through the examination criteria and procedures together.
2 Listen to the tape together.
3 Chart the information on the tape. Please will the examiners do this as well. Compare your charts to the example charts.
4 Ensure that you have been in contact with your regional organiser.

Charting for the Dental Examination (PLEASE CHART IN PENCIL)
It is important in large scale national surveys that as much comparability of method is achieved as possible. This reduces to a minimum slight variations of techniques between different examining and recording teams. It also facilitates coping with any emergency such as illness if a substitute dentist or recorder is trained on exactly the same methods.

If possible the recorder should sit so that the examiner can see the form and be reminded of the order of examination. The recorder should also use some headings as prompts. This serves two purposes both to remind the dentist of the next part of the examination and to tell the dentist that the recorder is ready to go on. The prompts used need to be discreet as they should not cause any concern to the children, and are suggested in the examples. The information is called out, in code, by the dentist so as again to avoid concern among the children. The examination chart has been

designed so that one form can be used whatever the age of the child and this has some consequences for the first section.

Order for examination

The examination is conducted in the order upper left – upper right – lower right – lower left. This order is kept to consistently throughout the examination.

Tooth type

The first thing that must be ascertained is what tooth type is under scrutiny. We need to establish for each possible tooth position whether it is the deciduous or permanent dentition that we are concerned with. The dentist looks at the child's mouth and calls out which he is concerned with giving the tooth number or letter as appropriate. If both the deciduous and permanent tooth are present then ring both the letter and the number (the dentist will later give the condition of the permanent tooth only).

Surfaces

When the dentist has identified the teeth he will then assess the condition of the surfaces. He will examine all five surfaces (or four for anterior teeth). He will do this in a given order and so he will not need to say the surface name but only the five (or four) codes in order, and you would enter one in each of the boxes provided. There are some conditions which involve the *whole tooth* and need only therefore be recorded in the first box, for example tooth unerupted (U), tooth extracted for caries (M), tooth missing due to trauma (T), or tooth extracted for orthodontic reasons (O).

The codes that can affect *surfaces* of a tooth differently are caries free (G), filled (F), decayed (code 2), unrestorable (code 3) and filled and decayed (code 4). Although these may occur in any combination for a particular tooth it will often be the case that the tooth is wholly caries free. In this case the dentist can say "All

G" after the tooth number. The recorder will then enter G in the first box and run a line down through two or three of the remaining boxes (see example). If the dentist is calling out a condition involving decay he should say 'code 2' or 'code 3' or 'code 4' rather than just the number so that the code number does not get confused with a tooth number.

The dentist should pause slightly at the mid-line point of the examination to make sure that the recorder has not been left behind and to ensure that the central teeth are properly distinguished one from the other.

Because it is unlikely that the children examined will have any 'eights', the 'eights' have been pre-coded U (unerupted) on the exam chart. If, however, a child has such a tooth present the appropriate code should be overwritten.

If the dentist or recorder makes a mistake the examination must stop immediately and start again at the last known point of agreement. It will be fairly obvious when the dentist wants to make such a break but the recorder will have to shout out to stop the flow of the dentist. It is much better to stop the dentist as soon as possible and then less has to be re-done.

If the dentist wants to make a special note of something he will say "asterisk" and the recorder will put an asterisk at that point of the examination. At the end of the exam (13) she will ring code 1 if he has called out an asterisk or ask him if he has any comments to make and if so ring code 1. Otherwise she will ring code O. If a code 1 has been ringed she will give the dentist the form so that he can write his comments down.

Examples of charts and a tape are enclosed

The examples of charting give illustrations of the above points which are much easier to absorb from practice than from description.

SURVEY OF CHILD DENTAL HEALTH

1983

THE CONDUCT OF THE EXAMINATION

AND CRITERIA FOR THE

ASSESSMENTS

Office of Population Censuses and Surveys

Department of Dental Health
University of Birmingham

Department of Child Dental Health
University of Newcastle upon Tyne

RACIAL ORIGIN

The racial origin of the child will be recorded. This may not be the same as the nationality or country of birth. There is considerable variation between individuals of the same race, especially in skin colour. Classification is to be assessed by physical appearance only.

White/Caucasion (Code 1)

Only those of 'white' European origin are recorded in this category. Individuals have a 'white' skin and fair, brown, red or black hair, which may be wavy or straight.

Negro (Code 2)

These individuals have a dark ('black') skin and black woolly hair.

Indian/Pakistani (Code 3)

Features include a light brown skin, black straight hair and a narrow nose.

Oriental (Code 4)

These have a 'yellow' skin, black coarse straight hair and a low bridge of the nose; the eyes often slant and the cheekbones are prominent.

Other (Code 5)

Specify any individual who can be classified into a racial group other than those above.

Not known (Code 6)

This category is to be used when the examiner is unable to classify the subject into any racial group.

1. TOOTH CONDITION

Teeth will be examined in the following order:

>   Upper left - upper right - lower right - lower left.

Tooth type

In the first instance the teeth will be identified and recorded. If a primary tooth is missing, always record the state of the permanent successor. In cases where both the primary tooth and its permanent successor are present, both will be identified and called but further details will be recorded for the permanent tooth only.

A tooth is deemed to be present if any part of it is visible. Permanent teeth may be absent for a number of reasons, as follows:

Code U   Unerupted

Code M   Extracted due to caries

Code T   Missing due to trauma

Code O   Extracted for orthodontic reasons

In most cases the reason for the absence of a permanent tooth will be obvious and the appropriate code may be called and recorded at once. Sometimes questioning the child will be necessary - "Did you have those teeth taken out to make room for the others?" "Was that front tooth knocked out?"

Tooth surfaces

If a tooth is present each surface will be examined, coded and called in the following order:

>   Mesial - occlusal - distal - buccal - lingual.

>   (In the cases of anterior teeth 'occlusal' is, of course, omitted.)

Surfaces obscured (eg by an orthodontic band) will be assumed to be sound unless there is clear evidence to the contrary.

N.B.   WHERE DOUBT EXISTS IN THE DIFFERENTIATION BETWEEN THE CATEGORIES, THE LESS SEVERE CATEGORY SHOULD ALWAYS BE CALLED.

The surface coding is as follows:

Code G   Present

In the case of partly-erupted teeth, where some surfaces may not be visible, these will be considered as sound and called under this category. Traumatised teeth, including those with permanent or semi-permanent restorations following fracture will also be coded in this category. The code G is thus used for all surfaces that are present and have had no caries experience.

Code F   Filled

Surfaces containing a permanent restoration of any material, will be coded under this category. Lesions or cavities containing a temporary dressing, or cavities from which a restoration has been lost, will be coded in the appropriate category of 'decayed'.

Code 2   Decayed

Surfaces are regarded as decayed if, in the opinion of the examiner, after visual inspection, there is a carious cavity that does not involve the pulp. If doubt exists the surface will be investigated with the probe supplied and unless the point enters the lesion the surface will be recorded as sound (G). The catching of the probe in a pit or fissure is not enough to warrant the diagnosis of caries unless there is additional visual evidence of it.

Code 3   Unrestorable

Surfaces are regarded as falling into this category if, in the opinion of the examiner, after scrutiny and testing as above, there is a carious cavity that involves the pulp. (The cavity that necessitates extraction or pulp treatment.)

Code 4   Filled and decayed

A surface that has a filling and a carious lesion will fall into this category unless the carious lesion would be coded as 'unrestorable', in which case the filling will be ignored and the surface classified as Code 3.

Communication of Codes to the Recorder

When calling out codes the names of the surfaces should not be mentioned. Just state the tooth number and the surface codes in the correct order.

When calling alphabetic codes the letter alone may be used. When calling numeric codes the number must be preceded by the word 'code' - this will avoid confusion between code numbers and tooth numbers. Where all surfaces of a tooth are code G the dentist may call the tooth number followed by 'all G'.

2. FISSURE SEALANTS

The occlusal surfaces of the permanent molars and premolars will be examined with the probe and the presence of fissure sealants recorded as follows:

0   No sealants present in any teeth

1   Sealant present on part or all of any surface

2   Assessment cannot be made, there are no permanent molars or premolars present

If any sealant is present the treated teeth will be ringed on the appropriate part of the chart in the same sequence as before.

Fissure sealants can be difficult to detect. To confirm his assessment the examiner may ask the child whether his/her teeth have been sealed.

3. TRAUMA OF PERMANENT INCISORS

Upper and lower incisors will be examined for traumatic injury and recorded as follows:

0   No trauma exists in any of these teeth

1   Trauma exists in one or more teeth

2   Assessment cannot be made, there are no permanent incisors present

If there is injury to any incisor then identify the teeth involved and code one or more of the following categories for each affected tooth.

1   Discolouration
2   Fracture involving enamel
3   "   "   enamel and dentine
4   "   "   enamel, dentine and pulp
5   Missing due to trauma
6   Acid-etch composite restoration
7   Permanent crown including jacket and post crowns, whether porcelain or acrylic
8   Other permanent or semi-permanent restorations. This refers to items of treatment such as stainless steel crowns, pinch bands, cellulose acetate crowns, Directa crowns, pinned inlays, etc.
9   Denture provided due to traumatic loss of this tooth

118

4. PERIO I

Gums, debris, calculus (all children)

For these assessments each jaw is divided into three segments, as follows:

The middle segment: extending forwards from the distal surface of the canine on one side around to the distal surface of the canine on the other side.

The left and right segments: extending backwards from the distal surfaces of the canines to the distal surfaces of the most posterior teeth present.

The examiner will look at each of these segments in the prescribed order (upper left, upper middle, upper right, lower right, lower middle, lower left) three times; once for the assessment of the gum condition, once for estimating the amount of debris on the teeth and once to determine the presence or absence of calculus. The average condition of the gums or debris in the segment should be recorded and not the worst area in that segment.

IT MUST BE STRESSED THAT WHEN THERE IS DOUBT ABOUT THE CLASSIFICATION OF ANY CONDITION, THE LOWER CATEGORY SHOULD BE RECORDED.

Gums:

Each segment will be examined both buccally and lingually and its state recorded according to one of the following categories:

0   The gums appear healthy. No treatment is needed.

1   The gums are not healthy. The condition is reversible; treatment in the form of prophylaxis and the correction of oral hygiene should restore them to health.

2   There is considerable redness and swelling of the gums. The condition is irreversible and the patient cannot be restored to health without the intervention of a dental surgeon involving possible surgery, extraction or replacement of faulty restorations.

Abscesses are ignored in assessing the gum condition, these should be noted with an asterisk and specified at the end of the examination under 'dentists comments'.

Debris: (Food material, materia alba, plaque)

Each segment will be examined visually both buccally and lingually and its state coded according to one of the following categories:

0   The teeth are clean. No debris is evident.

1   There is a small quantity of debris of recent origin. Ignore recent debris such as small pieces of potato crisp found in an otherwise clean mouth immediately following a school breaktime.

2   The teeth are dirty. There is considerable debris of long standing.

Calculus:

Each segment will be examined visually and the presence of calculus recorded as follows:

0   No calculus

1   Calculus is present

5. PERIO II

Pocketing and gingivitis (15 year olds only)

If child is aged 5-14 code 1 and go to occlusal assessment

Pocketing:

The assessment of pocketing will be made on the following permanent teeth:

    Upper left first molar

    Upper right central incisor

    Upper right first molar

    Lower right first molar

    Lower left central incisor

    Lower left first molar

If one, or more of the first molars are missing then the second molar(s) should be examined instead. If the upper right central incisor is missing, examine the upper left central incisor. If the lower left central incisor is absent examine the lower right central incisor. If both upper central incisors, or both lower central incisors, or one of the substituted second molars are missing, the assessment should be abandoned for that particular segment, and a score of 9 recorded.

The examination should be carried out in the same sequence as before (upper left, upper middle, upper right, lower right, lower middle and lower left). The periodontal probe should be gently inserted into the sulcus or pocket on the distal of each designated tooth and run around the buccal sulcus of the upper tooth, and the lingual sulcus of the lower tooth, to the mesial surface. The deepest position of the gingival margin in relation to the markings on the probe should be recorded in the following way:

0   All of the black portion of the probe is visible

1   Only part of the black portion is visible

2   None of the black portion is visible

9   Not recordable

Gingivitis:

After completion of the examination for the presence or absence of pockets, the gingivae in relation to these teeth will be examined in the same sequence as previously, for any evidence of bleeding, recorded as:

0   No bleeding from the gingival sulcus

1   Bleeding from the gingival sulcus

9   Not recordable

If a score 9 has been recorded under pocketing for the designated tooth in a particular segment, score 9 for gingivitis in that segment also.

NO PROBE WILL BE USED ON A SECOND CHILD WITHOUT SATISFACTORY STERILISATION.

120

OCCLUSAL ASSESSMENT

If none of the permanent upper incisors is present, do not carry out the occlusal assessment. Record 'no permanent upper incisors present', and go to section 13.

6. OVERJET

If the upper left central incisor is absent, or insufficiently erupted, code as 'not assessed'.
If the overjet is positive, or the overjet is zero, enter '+' in the space provided. If the overjet is reversed, record '-'.
Measure the overjet, with the gauge supplied, at the centre of the incisal edge.
If the measurement falls between marks on the gauge, record the lower mark.
Make a similar assessment for the upper right central incisor.

7. ROTATIONS

Rotation exists if any of the permanent upper central or lateral incisors are rotated by 30 degrees or more as judged by the use of the gauge supplied. If none of the upper incisors is rotated record 'none'; otherwise record 'some'.

8a   INSTANDING UPPER INCISORS

An instanding incisor is defined as a permanent upper central or lateral incisor occluding lingually to an opposing lower tooth. If none of the upper incisors is instanding, record 'none'. If any upper incisor is instanding record 'some' and ring the teeth involved.

8b. EDGE TO EDGE UPPER INCISORS

An edge-to-edge relationship occurs when any part of the incisor edge of a permanent upper central or lateral incisor occludes on any part of the incisal edge of an opposing lower tooth.

If none of the upper incisors is edge-to-edge, then record 'none'. If any upper incisor is edge-to-edge, record 'some' and ring the teeth involved.

9. TRAUMATIC OVERBITE

The gingivae are considered to be damaged if they are ulcerated, or if there is evidence of gingival stripping associated with an increased overbite. Assess the anterior segments of the upper and the lower arch, on both the buccal and the lingual aspects. If there is no such damage record 'none'. If such damage exists record 'some'.

10. CROWDING

This is defined as insufficient space in the existing dental arch for the teeth to be accommodated without overlap or irregularity.

Potential crowding should be included (any teeth which are assumed to be unerupted should be included in the assessment). Teeth which are assumed to be congenitally missing should not be included in the assessment. Teeth which have been extracted for orthodontic reasons have already been recorded under 'tooth condition'.

Record each segment separately, the anterior segments include the incisors and canines, the left and the right segments include the premolars and molars.

When assessing the anterior segments, take account of any space that has been created immediately distal to the canine teeth, following the extraction of a premolar. For example, if lower first premolars have been extracted, and the extractions have created sufficient space for the alignment of all the teeth in the anterior segment, record the anterior segment as uncrowded.

Record in the following categories:

    0   No crowding, all the teeth present in this segment including those
         as yet unerupted can be fitted into the arch without overlap or
         irregularity

    1   The teeth in this segment of the arch are crowded

11. ORTHO APPLIANCES

If the child is not wearing an appliance, then ask whether or not he/she has worn one in the past.

If the child has never worn an appliance ring '1' and go to 12.

If the child is wearing an orthodontic appliance, record the fact on the examination form, and specify the type of appliance which is being worn. Use the following categories:

0   No appliance in this jaw

1   Removeable orthodontic appliance

2   Fixed orthodontic appliance

3   Other. In this case, describe the type of appliance in the section
     reserved for comments

If the child has worn an orthodontic appliance at some time, then ask whether he/she still wears the appliance, or whether the appliance treatment is finished.

122

12. ORTHO TREATMENT NEED

If the child is currently wearing an orthodontic appliance, record '1' and go to section 13.
If no orthodontic treatment is needed, record '0'.
If the child needs, or in your opinion will need, orthodontic treatment, then record '2'.
If child needs or will need orthodontic treatment, record which of the following occlusal features are likely to need treatment. You can specify more than one feature.

1   Overjet

2   Instanding incisor

3   Rotated incisor

4   Gingival trauma

5   Crowding

6   Other

If the child needs, or will need, orthodontic treatment for some occlusal anomaly which is not included in this list, record as 'other'. In this case make a note of the feature requiring correction, using the section of the examination form provided.

13. ASTERISK/COMMENTS (Instructions to the recorder)

At any time during the examination if the dentist wishes to make comments he will call 'asterisk' to the recorder who will mark the form at that point.

On completion of the examination, if there are no asterisks marked, ask if the dentist wishes to make a comment. If the dentist has no comment to make ring 'none'. If there are any asterisks and/or the dentist does wish to comment, ring 'some' and hand the examination form to the dentist to record comments on the back.

W2435G OPCS 11/82

Appendix D The dental team

Dental schools

University of Birmingham
Dr R J Anderson
Ms G Bradnock
Dr L Shaw
Professor P M C James

University of Newcastle upon Tyne
Professor J J Murray
Dr P H Gordon
Dr J H Nunn

Regional dental organisers
Dr J Beal
Mr R Bettles
Dr R J Elderton
Dr A French
Mr J Onions
Mr J Palmer
Mr J Rhodes
Mr N Whitehouse

The dentists

Mr L W J Anderson	Mr P Gore	Mr R Maxwell	Mrs P Spencer
Mrs M Attrill	Mr D Gorton	Mr M C Merrett	Mr D K Stables
Mr D Attwood	Mr G E Griffith	Mr G Morgan	Mrs M Stott
Mr P D Bainton	Mr P A Hancock	Mr J A E Morris	Mr A J Swan
Mr A Bewick	Mr D M Hobbs	Mr K J Moss	Mr G Taylor
Mr R Blankenstein	Mrs C P Hurst	Miss R C Nesbitt	Mr J F G Thomas
Mr H Breslin	Mr R J Izon	Mr J Newman	Miss P L Thompson
Mrs H V Burke	Mr P A Jenkins	Mr D R Pearse	Mrs F Thomson
Mr L S Campbell	Mr T P Johnston	Mr J P B Pengelly	Mr H J Trimlett
Mr A J Casey	Mr C W D Jones	Mr M J Prendegast	Mrs E Twyford
Miss M B Cogan	Mrs H M Kelly	Mr W A Quirk	Mr D Vaughan
Mr G Crawford	Mr J W Langford	Mr H R Rippon	Mrs E Vince
Mr J Cullen	Mr A J Lawrence	Mrs K H Rothwell	Mr R C Ward
Mrs E Davies	Ms P M Llewelyn	Miss R A Russell	Mr C A Wilkinson
Mr P G Davies	Mr T S Longworth	Miss E J Salisch	Mr M Williams
Mr R L Davies	Mr H D Lunn	Miss J S Sandham	Mr K Woods
Mr G J Derbyshire	Mr J W McConnachie	Mrs S M Saunders	Mr A Yardley
Mr M Dyer	Mrs R McMullin	Ms J Smith	Mr P Young
Mr W H Garland			

Appendix E Appendix tables

Appendix Table 1 Mean, standard deviation and percentage components of decayed, missing and filled deciduous and permanent teeth, by age and sex: United Kingdom and constituent countries

Age (years)	Deciduous teeth					Permanent teeth					
	Mean dft	St. Dev.	%d/dft	%f/dft	Base	Mean DMFT	St. Dev.	% D/DMFT	% M/DMFT	% F/DMFT	Base
United Kingdom											
Males											
5	1.9	2.551	72	28	423	–	0.150	100	–	–	423
6	2.1	2.639	63	37	421	0.1	0.439	60	–	40	421
7	2.5	2.596	55	45	487	0.4	0.919	45	1	55	487
8	2.4	2.244	51	49	500	0.8	1.241	39	4	56	500
9	2.3	2.098	49	51	549	1.2	1.523	29	7	65	549
10	1.9	1.940	45	55	609	1.7	1.793	29	7	64	609
11	1.3	1.787	45	55	614	2.3	2.138	25	9	66	614
12	0.5	1.080	54	46	598	3.0	2.625	22	10	68	598
13	0.2	0.570	46	54	631	3.8	3.310	21	9	70	631
14	0.1	0.400	34	66	651	4.7	3.601	20	7	73	651
15	–	0.175	47	53	586	5.8	3.929	17	10	73	586
Females											
5	1.7	2.495	71	29	381	–	0.135	90	–	10	381
6	2.0	2.506	64	36	442	0.1	0.544	61	2	37	442
7	2.3	2.542	54	46	434	0.4	0.891	50	3	48	434
8	2.3	2.337	49	51	468	0.9	1.341	34	6	60	468
9	2.2	2.145	44	56	512	1.4	1.602	28	7	65	512
10	1.5	1.782	43	57	543	1.8	1.765	24	8	68	543
11	1.0	1.447	43	57	563	2.5	2.361	23	9	68	563
12	0.4	0.875	44	56	567	3.2	2.621	19	9	72	567
13	0.1	0.498	43	57	561	4.1	3.231	17	10	73	561
14	0.1	0.328	43	57	597	5.1	3.703	17	9	74	597
15	–	0.211	36	64	571	6.1	3.927	15	10	75	571
Both sexes											
5	1.8	2.525	72	28	804	–	0.143	96	–	4	804
6	2.1	2.570	64	36	863	0.1	0.496	60	1	38	863
7	2.4	2.571	55	45	921	0.4	0.905	47	2	51	921
8	2.3	2.288	50	50	968	0.8	1.292	37	5	58	968
9	2.3	2.120	47	53	1,061	1.3	1.563	28	7	65	1,061
10	1.7	1.874	44	56	1,152	1.8	1.779	27	8	66	1,152
11	1.1	1.642	44	56	1,177	2.4	2.249	24	9	67	1,177
12	0.4	0.987	50	50	1,165	3.1	2.624	21	10	70	1,165
13	0.1	0.538	44	56	1,192	3.9	3.275	19	9	72	1,192
14	0.1	0.367	38	62	1,248	4.9	3.655	19	8	73	1,248
15	–	0.194	40	60	1,156	5.9	3.930	16	10	74	1,156
England and Wales											
Males											
5	1.7	2.423	70	30	378	–	0.126	100	–	–	378
6	2.0	2.566	62	38	373	0.1	0.405	60	–	40	373
7	2.4	2.589	54	46	439	0.3	0.867	40	–	60	439
8	2.3	2.214	49	51	446	0.7	1.155	40	4	57	446
9	2.3	2.104	48	52	495	1.1	1.450	27	6	66	495
10	1.9	1.956	44	56	553	1.7	1.746	28	7	65	553
11	1.3	1.819	43	57	550	2.1	1.983	24	8	68	550
12	0.5	1.099	54	46	531	2.8	2.517	21	10	69	531
13	0.2	0.569	43	57	569	3.6	3.216	20	8	72	569
14	0.1	0.409	33	67	581	4.5	3.429	19	6	75	581
15	–	0.180	46	54	527	5.5	3.768	16	9	75	527
Females											
5	1.5	2.284	69	31	341	–	0.121	90	–	10	341
6	1.9	2.455	63	37	397	0.1	0.521	61	2	36	397
7	2.2	2.504	53	47	390	0.4	0.804	48	3	49	390
8	2.2	2.309	47	53	419	0.8	1.280	33	6	61	419
9	2.2	2.148	43	57	463	1.3	1.543	26	7	67	463
10	1.5	1.785	42	58	493	1.6	1.678	23	8	69	493
11	1.0	1.455	42	58	508	2.3	2.287	23	9	68	508
12	0.4	0.888	43	57	505	3.0	2.422	18	9	74	505
13	0.1	0.497	41	59	493	3.8	3.014	16	9	75	493
14	0.1	0.336	42	58	528	4.9	3.488	17	8	75	528
15	–	0.208	31	69	510	5.8	3.687	15	9	76	510
Both sexes											
5	1.6	2.358	69	31	719	–	0.124	96	–	4	719
6	1.9	2.508	63	37	770	0.1	0.469	61	2	38	770
7	2.3	2.551	53	47	829	0.3	0.838	44	1	55	829
8	2.2	2.259	48	52	865	0.7	1.219	36	5	59	865
9	2.2	2.124	46	54	957	1.2	1.497	27	7	66	957
10	1.7	1.884	43	57	1,046	1.7	1.713	26	7	67	1,046
11	1.2	1.663	43	57	1,058	2.2	2.136	24	8	68	1,058
12	0.4	1.003	49	51	1,036	2.9	2.472	19	9	71	1,036
13	0.2	0.537	42	58	1,062	3.7	3.124	18	9	73	1,062
14	0.1	0.376	37	63	1,109	4.7	3.461	18	7	75	1,109
15	–	0.195	37	63	1,038	5.6	3.730	16	9	75	1,038

Appendix Table 1 *continued*

Age (years)	Deciduous teeth					Permanent teeth					
	Mean dft	St. Dev.	%d/dft	%f/dft	*Base*	Mean DMFT	St. Dev.	% D/DMFT	% M/DMFT	% F/DMFT	*Base*
England											
Males											
5	1.7	2.368	70	30	*351*	–	0.130	100	–	–	*351*
6	1.9	2.549	63	37	*349*	0.1	0.407	61	–	39	*349*
7	2.4	2.584	53	47	*410*	0.3	0.870	40	–	60	*410*
8	2.2	2.196	48	52	*417*	0.7	1.145	40	4	56	*417*
9	2.2	2.084	47	53	*462*	1.1	1.453	27	7	66	*462*
10	1.9	1.946	43	57	*519*	1.7	1.757	29	7	65	*519*
11	1.3	1.836	42	58	*515*	2.1	1.961	24	8	69	*515*
12	0.5	1.094	52	48	*496*	2.8	2.525	21	10	69	*496*
13	0.2	0.535	42	58	*533*	3.5	3.176	19	8	73	*533*
14	0.1	0.417	32	68	*543*	4.4	3.408	19	6	76	*543*
15	–	0.185	–	–	*493*	5.4	3.717	16	8	75	*493*
Females											
5	1.5	2.221	69	31	*320*	–	0.112	100	–	–	*320*
6	1.9	2.388	62	38	*368*	0.1	0.523	61	2	37	*368*
7	2.2	2.513	53	47	*362*	0.4	0.809	48	3	49	*362*
8	2.2	2.313	46	54	*394*	0.8	1.273	33	6	61	*394*
9	2.2	2.150	43	57	*429*	1.3	1.550	26	7	67	*429*
10	1.5	1.791	42	58	*464*	1.6	1.649	23	8	69	*464*
11	1.0	1.441	42	58	*474*	2.3	2.286	23	9	69	*474*
12	0.4	0.897	43	57	*475*	2.9	2.421	18	8	74	*475*
13	0.1	0.497	39	61	*458*	3.7	3.987	16	9	75	*458*
14	0.1	0.341	44	56	*499*	4.8	3.466	17	8	75	*499*
15	–	0.214	–	–	*474*	5.7	3.636	15	9	76	*474*
Both sexes											
5	1.6	2.299	69	31	*671*	–	0.122	100	–	–	*671*
6	1.9	2.466	63	37	*717*	0.1	0.471	61	1	38	*717*
7	2.3	2.551	53	47	*772*	0.4	0.842	44	1	55	*772*
8	2.2	2.252	47	53	*811*	0.7	1.210	37	5	58	*811*
9	2.2	2.115	45	55	*891*	1.2	1.502	27	7	66	*891*
10	1.7	1.880	43	57	*983*	1.6	1.706	26	7	67	*983*
11	1.2	1.668	42	58	*989*	2.2	2.126	23	8	69	*989*
12	0.4	1.003	48	52	*971*	2.9	2.475	19	9	72	*971*
13	0.1	0.518	41	59	*991*	3.6	3.090	18	9	74	*991*
14	0.1	0.383	37	63	*1,042*	4.6	3.441	18	7	75	*1,042*
15	–	0.200	–	–	*967*	5.6	3.678	15	9	76	*967*
Wales											
Males											
5	2.7	2.908	70	30	*107*	–	–	–	–	–	*107*
6	2.8	2.653	55	45	*96*	0.1	0.363	43	–	57	*96*
7	2.8	2.654	62	38	*116*	0.3	0.833	38	–	62	*116*
8	3.0	2.339	55	45	*116*	0.9	1.289	31	6	63	*116*
9	3.0	2.250	54	46	*129*	1.2	1.398	29	4	67	*129*
10	2.2	2.091	52	48	*133*	1.6	1.580	21	4	75	*133*
11	1.0	1.532	51	49	*139*	2.7	2.199	32	10	58	*139*
12	0.6	1.166	71	29	*138*	3.3	2.365	19	10	71	*138*
13	0.3	0.940	55	45	*141*	4.4	3.675	24	11	65	*141*
14	–	0.244	80	20	*149*	5.6	3.553	25	9	67	*149*
15	–	0.086	100	–	*136*	6.7	4.273	19	12	70	*136*
Females											
5	2.4	2.964	69	31	*83*	–	0.220	50	–	50	*83*
6	2.5	3.144	71	29	*115*	0.1	0.498	64	7	29	*115*
7	2.1	2.401	55	45	*109*	0.2	0.715	60	–	40	*109*
8	2.5	2.232	54	46	*97*	1.0	1.392	25	3	72	*97*
9	2.3	2.118	52	48	*133*	1.3	1.464	29	5	66	*133*
10	1.5	1.697	42	58	*116*	2.0	2.066	25	13	63	*116*
11	1.0	1.637	48	52	*133*	2.5	2.305	29	9	62	*133*
12	0.3	0.735	50	50	*120*	3.4	2.414	21	11	68	*120*
13	0.1	0.492	61	39	*140*	4.5	3.255	19	11	70	*140*
14	–	0.227	–	100	*115*	5.6	3.785	13	11	76	*115*
15	–	0.118	100	–	*143*	6.7	4.219	16	11	73	*143*
Both sexes											
5	2.6	2.927	69	31	*190*	–	0.145	50	–	50	*190*
6	2.7	2.929	63	37	*211*	0.1	0.441	57	5	38	*211*
7	2.4	2.549	59	41	*225*	0.3	0.779	47	–	53	*225*
8	2.8	2.295	54	46	*213*	0.9	1.335	28	5	67	*213*
9	2.7	2.205	53	47	*262*	1.3	1.430	29	4	67	*262*
10	1.9	1.942	48	52	*249*	1.8	1.827	23	9	69	*249*
11	1.0	1.581	50	50	*272*	2.6	2.250	31	10	60	*272*
12	0.5	1.002	65	35	*258*	3.3	2.384	20	10	70	*258*
13	0.2	0.753	57	43	*281*	4.5	3.467	21	11	68	*281*
14	–	0.236	44	56	*264*	5.6	3.649	19	10	71	*264*
15	–	0.103	100	–	*279*	6.7	4.237	17	11	71	*279*

Age (years)	Deciduous teeth					Permanent teeth					
	Mean dft	St. Dev.	%d/dft	%f/dft	*Base*	Mean DMFT	St. Dev.	% D/DMFT	% M/DMFT	% F/DMFT	*Base*
Scotland											
Males											
5	3.3	2.921	84	16	*172*	–	0.263	100	–	–	*172*
6	3.4	2.982	69	31	*176*	0.2	0.596	66	–	34	*176*
7	2.9	2.569	65	35	*182*	0.6	1.153	63	5	32	*182*
8	3.4	2.330	63	37	*221*	1.4	1.513	42	5	53	*221*
9	2.6	2.084	60	40	*208*	2.1	1.855	33	11	56	*208*
10	1.8	1.771	57	43	*224*	2.4	2.002	24	9	57	*224*
11	1.0	1.444	65	35	*259*	3.6	2.951	29	11	60	*259*
12	0.5	0.905	57	43	*278*	4.3	3.224	27	12	61	*278*
13	0.2	0.599	70	30	*253*	5.6	3.602	28	12	60	*253*
14	–	0.344	50	50	*300*	6.5	4.098	26	15	58	*300*
15	–	0.064	–	100	*246*	8.2	4.436	22	14	64	*246*
Females											
5	3.2	3.409	79	21	*147*	–	0.116	100	–	–	*147*
6	3.0	2.781	64	36	*181*	0.2	0.615	58	–	42	*181*
7	3.2	2.554	63	37	*175*	0.9	1.283	52	1	48	*175*
8	3.1	2.498	60	40	*191*	1.7	1.597	38	7	56	*191*
9	2.3	2.143	51	49	*193*	2.0	1.821	33	6	62	*193*
10	1.4	1.741	54	46	*192*	2.9	2.113	26	12	62	*192*
11	0.8	1.430	54	46	*220*	3.6	2.495	20	9	70	*220*
12	0.3	0.754	52	48	*247*	4.8	3.468	21	13	66	*247*
13	0.1	0.508	52	48	*254*	6.1	3.642	18	12	70	*254*
14	–	0.268	45	55	*288*	7.1	4.411	18	13	69	*288*
15	–	0.246	64	36	*240*	8.8	4.712	14	13	73	*240*
Both sexes											
5	3.2	3.151	81	19	*319*	–	0.208	100	–	–	*319*
6	3.2	2.883	67	33	*357*	0.2	0.605	61	–	39	*357*
7	3.0	2.563	64	36	*357*	0.8	1.226	56	3	41	*357*
8	3.3	2.409	62	38	*412*	1.5	1.556	40	6	54	*412*
9	2.5	2.113	56	44	*401*	2.1	1.837	33	8	59	*401*
10	1.6	1.765	55	45	*416*	2.7	2.064	30	11	60	*416*
11	0.9	1.440	60	40	*479*	3.6	2.748	25	10	65	*479*
12	0.4	0.841	55	45	*525*	4.5	3.347	24	13	64	*525*
13	0.1	0.557	65	35	*507*	5.9	3.627	23	12	65	*507*
14	–	0.309	48	52	*588*	6.8	4.258	22	14	64	*588*
15	–	0.180	58	42	*486*	8.4	4.579	18	14	68	*486*
Northern Ireland											
Males											
5	3.8	3.315	80	20	*99*	–	0.317	100	–	–	*99*
6	2.9	2.782	73	27	*113*	0.3	0.718	56	–	44	*113*
7	3.4	2.650	73	27	*109*	1.0	1.404	66	1	33	*109*
8	3.1	2.040	59	41	*96*	2.1	1.763	33	7	61	*96*
9	2.3	1.906	59	41	*123*	2.3	1.733	35	6	59	*123*
10	2.1	1.810	64	36	*116*	2.9	2.041	36	11	53	*116*
11	1.3	1.529	61	39	*123*	3.6	2.516	30	13	56	*123*
12	0.5	0.969	73	27	*120*	4.3	2.410	28	18	54	*120*
13	0.2	0.534	58	42	*120*	5.6	3.461	33	15	52	*120*
14	–	0.186	50	50	*113*	7.4	4.930	24	12	63	*113*
15	–	0.227	100	–	*96*	8.7	4.427	26	17	57	*96*
Females											
5	3.6	3.599	80	20	*99*	0.1	0.340	88	–	13	*99*
6	3.0	2.615	72	28	*89*	0.3	0.929	57	–	43	*89*
7	3.7	2.834	67	33	*92*	1.1	1.422	57	5	38	*92*
8	2.8	2.325	62	38	*106*	1.7	1.571	44	8	47	*106*
9	2.5	2.043	55	45	*102*	2.9	1.815	38	11	51	*102*
10	1.9	1.755	60	40	*108*	3.4	1.971	35	9	56	*108*
11	0.6	1.121	40	60	*110*	4.4	2.882	34	15	51	*110*
12	0.3	0.744	66	34	*119*	5.3	3.318	35	13	53	*119*
13	0.1	0.515	76	24	*156*	7.0	4.066	25	14	61	*156*
14	–	0.228	75	25	*114*	8.0	4.904	20	13	67	*114*
15	–	0.182	100	–	*121*	9.6	4.497	21	12	67	*121*
Both sexes											
5	3.7	3.453	80	20	*198*	0.1	0.329	92	–	8	*198*
6	3.0	2.703	72	28	*202*	0.3	0.816	56	–	44	*202*
7	3.5	2.733	70	30	*201*	1.0	1.410	62	3	35	*201*
8	3.0	2.193	61	39	*202*	1.9	1.673	38	8	54	*202*
9	2.4	1.967	57	43	*225*	2.5	1.790	36	8	55	*225*
10	2.0	1.781	62	38	*224*	3.1	2.018	35	10	54	*224*
11	0.9	1.396	55	45	*233*	3.9	2.718	32	14	54	*233*
12	0.4	0.868	70	30	*239*	4.8	2.935	32	15	53	*239*
13	0.1	0.523	67	33	*276*	6.4	3.871	28	14	57	*276*
14	–	0.207	63	38	*227*	7.7	4.915	22	13	65	*227*
15	–	0.203	100	–	*217*	9.2	4.478	23	14	63	*217*

Appendix Table 2 Mean, standard deviation and percentage components of decayed, missing and filled deciduous and permanent teeth, by age: Regional Health Areas

Age (years)	Deciduous teeth					Permanent teeth					
	Mean dft	St. Dev.	%d/dft	%f/dft	Base	Mean DMFT	St. Dev.	% D/DMFT	% M/DMFT	% F/DMFT	Base
North West											
5	2.1	2.635	72	28	100	–	–	–	–	–	100
6	2.5	2.570	69	31	109	0.1	0.621	75	–	25	109
7	3.4	2.793	59	41	109	0.6	1.089	65	–	35	109
8	2.8	2.399	55	45	120	1.0	1.375	41	9	50	120
9	2.6	2.158	56	44	138	1.6	1.733	33	9	58	138
10	2.0	1.897	56	44	163	2.3	1.876	34	13	53	163
11	1.1	1.608	57	43	150	3.0	2.275	29	11	60	150
12	0.5	1.061	64	36	147	3.9	3.005	28	12	59	147
13	0.1	0.403	57	43	140	5.1	3.691	22	13	66	140
14	–	0.163	25	75	147	5.7	3.354	20	8	71	147
15	–	0.222	60	40	139	6.6	3.893	21	11	68	139
North and North East											
5	1.3	2.056	75	25	121	–	0.182	100	–	–	121
6	1.7	2.214	65	35	123	0.2	0.657	52	–	48	123
7	2.2	2.195	54	46	136	0.5	1.046	31	–	69	136
8	1.8	1.903	58	42	140	0.8	1.253	50	7	44	140
9	2.0	1.824	51	49	185	1.3	1.502	19	12	69	185
10	1.6	1.605	48	52	165	1.7	1.619	22	16	63	165
11	0.9	1.369	42	58	177	2.1	2.022	21	15	64	177
12	0.5	0.988	58	42	172	2.8	2.406	14	12	74	172
13	0.1	0.496	64	36	168	3.4	2.799	14	16	71	168
14	–	0.216	25	75	209	4.5	3.415	11	8	80	209
15	–	0.123	67	33	195	6.1	3.709	15	13	73	195
West Midlands											
5	1.9	2.626	67	33	72	–	0.262	100	–	–	72
6	1.8	2.622	70	30	79	0.1	0.221	25	–	75	79
7	2.4	2.449	53	47	103	0.3	0.785	60	–	44	103
8	2.1	2.304	44	56	125	0.8	1.312	39	–	61	125
9	2.0	1.874	43	57	128	1.4	1.606	35	7	58	128
10	1.8	1.942	40	60	164	1.8	1.865	26	1	73	164
11	1.4	1.851	45	55	132	2.4	2.148	21	3	76	132
12	0.4	0.838	55	45	107	2.9	2.513	20	9	70	107
13	0.1	0.477	37	63	134	3.9	3.104	19	7	74	134
14	0.1	0.501	29	71	140	4.8	3.442	21	8	71	140
15	–	0.291	–	100	129	5.3	3.292	12	5	84	129
East Midlands											
5	1.5	2.258	60	40	79	–	0.113	100	–	–	79
6	1.7	2.266	43	57	77	0.1	0.531	18	9	73	77
7	1.7	2.295	40	60	96	0.2	0.661	30	–	70	96
8	2.0	2.162	45	55	93	0.6	1.101	20	–	80	93
9	1.6	1.981	46	54	91	0.8	1.405	15	4	80	91
10	1.5	1.712	44	56	95	1.4	1.724	18	5	77	95
11	1.0	1.380	39	61	107	1.9	1.750	22	6	71	107
12	0.4	0.839	43	57	126	2.4	2.236	18	7	75	126
13	0.1	0.526	42	58	97	3.0	2.642	14	2	85	97
14	0.1	0.503	62	38	118	3.8	3.423	19	9	72	118
15	–	0.098	100	–	104	4.5	3.367	10	9	81	104
South West											
5	1.2	2.041	66	34	78	–	–	–	–	–	78
6	1.6	2.471	52	48	80	0.1	0.528	100	–	–	80
7	2.0	2.544	51	49	103	0.2	0.757	42	17	42	103
8	2.3	2.212	50	50	100	0.6	1.016	46	8	46	100
9	2.3	2.151	44	56	117	0.9	1.284	29	7	64	117
10	1.9	2.061	37	63	121	1.5	1.618	23	4	73	121
11	1.3	1.712	36	64	133	2.3	2.424	23	6	71	133
12	0.5	1.137	32	68	126	3.0	2.248	18	6	76	126
13	0.2	0.557	39	61	133	3.3	2.988	15	6	79	133
14	0.1	0.508	36	64	143	4.3	3.331	17	3	80	143
15	–	0.300	20	80	121	6.3	4.036	12	7	81	121
North Thames											
5	1.7	2.326	69	31	105	–	–	–	–	–	105
6	2.0	2.478	64	36	107	0.1	0.311	89	–	11	107
7	2.3	2.879	61	39	103	0.2	0.616	33	–	67	103
8	2.2	2.363	44	56	109	0.6	1.074	33	2	65	109
9	2.7	2.606	46	54	97	0.9	1.182	33	–	67	97
10	1.5	1.939	40	60	111	1.2	1.468	27	–	73	111
11	1.1	1.759	47	53	143	1.7	1.724	37	6	58	143
12	0.4	0.979	48	52	144	2.5	2.278	23	7	70	144
13	0.2	0.513	39	61	151	2.9	2.575	25	6	69	151
14	0.1	0.434	17	83	133	4.5	3.392	27	6	68	133
15	–	0.080	100	–	156	4.2	3.014	27	5	68	156
South Thames											
5	1.4	2.123	71	29	116	–	–	–	–	–	116
6	1.7	2.557	63	37	142	–	0.185	60	–	40	142
7	2.0	2.435	44	56	122	0.2	0.647	33	–	67	122
8	2.3	2.336	33	67	124	0.7	1.198	20	7	73	124
9	2.4	2.215	26	74	135	1.0	1.438	16	–	84	135
10	1.8	1.950	31	69	164	1.3	1.411	24	3	73	164
11	1.4	1.891	31	69	147	2.0	2.180	11	5	84	147
12	0.4	1.105	35	65	149	2.5	2.259	12	7	81	149
13	0.2	0.615	24	76	168	3.6	3.154	14	5	81	168
14	0.1	0.277	63	38	152	4.3	3.510	12	5	84	152
15	–	0.201	–	100	123	5.7	3.715	10	9	81	123

Number of deciduous teeth	Age (years)										
	5	6	7	8	9	10	11	12	13	14	15
	%	%	%	%	%	%	%	%	%	%	%
United Kingdom											
Decayed (d)											
0	59	55	53	51	50	60	72	86	95	98	99
1	12	16	15	19	21	19	14	9	4	2	1
2	9	10	12	13	14	11	9	3	1	–	–
3	6	5	8	9	7	6	3	1	–	–	–
4	5	4	5	4	5	3	1	1	–	–	–
5	2	4	3	2	2	1	1	–	–	–	–
6	2	3	2	1	1	–	–	–	–	–	–
7	2	1	1	1	–	–	–	–	–	–	–
8	1	1	1	–	–	–	–	–	–	–	–
9	1	–	–	–	–	–	–	–	–	–	–
10	–	–	–	–	–	–	–	–	–	–	–
11 or more	–	–	–	–	–	–	–	–	–	–	–
Total	100	100	100	100	100	100	100	100	100	100	100
Mean	**1.3**	**1.3**	**1.3**	**1.2**	**1.1**	**0.8**	**0.5**	**0.2**	**0.1**	**–**	**–**
Filled (f)											
0	77	69	60	53	51	57	69	87	94	97	99
1	9	11	11	17	17	18	13	7	4	2	1
2	6	7	10	12	13	10	8	3	1	1	–
3	4	5	7	7	8	7	5	1	–	–	–
4	3	4	6	5	6	4	2	–	–	–	–
5	1	2	3	3	3	2	1	–	–	–	–
6	1	1	1	2	1	1	1	–	–	–	–
7	–	–	1	1	–	–	–	–	–	–	–
8 or more	–	–	–	–	–	–	–	–	–	–	–
Total	100	100	100	100	100	100	100	100	100	100	100
Mean	**0.5**	**0.8**	**1.1**	**1.2**	**1.2**	**1.0**	**0.6**	**0.2**	**0.1**	**–**	**–**
Decayed (d) + filled (f)											
0	49	44	36	30	29	38	55	77	91	96	98
1	12	12	11	15	15	17	15	12	6	3	1
2	9	10	12	14	17	15	12	6	2	1	–
3	7	8	10	13	12	12	7	2	1	–	–
4	8	9	10	9	11	8	5	1	–	–	–
5	4	6	9	8	9	5	3	1	–	–	–
6	4	5	5	6	5	3	2	–	–	–	–
7	3	2	3	4	2	1	1	–	–	–	–
8	2	3	2	1	1	1	–	–	–	–	–
9	1	1	1	1	–	–	–	–	–	–	–
10	–	1	1	–	–	–	–	–	–	–	–
11 or more	–	–	–	–	–	–	–	–	–	–	–
Total	100	100	100	100	100	100	100	100	100	100	100
Mean	**1.8**	**2.1**	**2.4**	**2.3**	**2.3**	**1.7**	**1.1**	**0.4**	**0.1**	**0.1**	**–**
Base	*804*	*863*	*921*	*968*	*1,061*	*1,152*	*1,177*	*1,165*	*1,192*	*1,248*	*1,156*
England and Wales											
Decayed (d)											
0	62	57	55	53	51	61	72	86	95	98	99
1	12	16	15	19	21	18	14	9	4	2	1
2	9	10	11	12	14	11	9	3	1	–	–
3	6	5	7	8	6	6	3	1	–	–	–
4	4	4	4	4	5	3	1	1	–	–	–
5	1	3	2	2	1	1	1	–	–	–	–
6	2	3	2	1	1	–	–	–	–	–	–
7	1	1	1	1	–	–	–	–	–	–	–
8	1	1	1	–	–	–	–	–	–	–	–
9	–	–	–	–	–	–	–	–	–	–	–
10	–	–	1	–	–	–	–	–	–	–	–
11 or more	–	–	–	–	–	–	–	–	–	–	–
Total	100	100	100	100	100	100	100	100	100	100	100
Mean	**1.1**	**1.2**	**1.2**	**1.1**	**1.0**	**0.7**	**0.5**	**0.2**	**0.1**	**–**	**–**
Filled (f)											
0	77	70	60	53	50	57	68	87	94	97	99
1	10	10	11	17	17	18	14	8	4	2	1
2	6	7	10	12	14	10	8	4	1	1	–
3	4	5	7	6	8	7	5	2	–	–	–
4	3	4	6	5	6	4	2	–	–	–	–
5	–	2	3	3	3	2	1	–	–	–	–
6	1	1	1	2	1	1	1	–	–	–	–
7	–	–	1	1	1	1	–	–	–	–	–
8 or more	–	–	–	–	–	–	–	–	–	–	–
	–	–	–	–	–	–	–	–	–	–	–
	–	–	–	–	–	–	–	–	–	–	–
Total	100	100	100	100	100	100	100	100	100	100	100
Mean	**0.5**	**0.7**	**1.1**	**1.2**	**1.2**	**1.0**	**0.7**	**0.2**	**0.1**	**–**	**–**

Number of deciduous teeth	Age (years)										
	5	6	7	8	9	10	11	12	13	14	15
	%	%	%	%	%	%	%	%	%	%	%
England and Wales *continued*											
Decayed (d) + filled (f)											
0	52	46	38	32	29	38	54	77	90	95	98
1	13	12	11	15	15	17	15	12	6	3	1
2	9	9	12	14	16	15	12	6	2	1	–
3	7	8	10	12	12	13	7	3	1	–	–
4	8	8	9	10	8	5	1	–	–	–	–
5	4	6	9	7	9	5	3	1	–	–	–
6	3	5	4	5	4	3	2	–	–	–	–
7	2	1	3	3	2	1	1	–	–	–	–
8	1	3	2	1	1	1	–	–	–	–	–
9	1	–	1	1	–	–	–	–	–	–	–
10	–	1	1	–	–	–	–	–	–	–	–
11 or more	–	–	–	–	–	–	–	–	–	–	–
Total	100	100	100	100	100	100	100	100	100	100	100
Mean	**1.6**	**1.9**	**2.3**	**2.2**	**2.2**	**1.7**	**1.2**	**0.4**	**0.2**	**0.1**	**–**
Base	719	770	829	865	957	1,046	1,058	1,036	1,062	1,109	1,038
England											
Decayed (d)											
0	63	57	56	54	52	62	72	87	95	98	99
1	12	16	15	19	21	18	14	9	3	2	1
2	9	9	12	12	14	11	9	2	1	–	–
3	6	4	7	8	6	5	3	1	–	–	–
4	4	4	4	3	4	3	1	1	–	–	–
5	1	3	2	2	1	1	1	–	–	–	–
6	2	3	2	1	1	–	–	–	–	–	–
7	1	1	1	1	–	–	–	–	–	–	–
8	1	1	1	–	–	–	–	–	–	–	–
9	–	–	–	–	–	–	–	–	–	–	–
10	–	–	1	–	–	–	–	–	–	–	–
11 or more	–	–	–	–	–	–	–	–	–	–	–
Total	100	100	100	100	100	100	100	100	100	100	100
Mean	**1.1**	**1.2**	**1.2**	**1.0**	**1.0**	**0.7**	**0.5**	**0.2**	**0.1**	**–**	**–**
Filled (f)											
0	78	71	60	54	50	56	68	86	94	97	99
1	9	10	10	17	18	18	14	8	4	2	1
2	5	7	10	12	13	10	8	4	2	1	–
3	4	5	7	6	8	7	5	2	1	–	–
4	3	3	6	5	6	4	2	1	–	–	–
5	–	2	3	3	3	2	1	–	–	–	–
6	1	1	1	2	1	1	1	–	–	–	–
7	–	–	1	1	1	1	–	–	–	–	–
8 or more	–	–	–	–	–	–	–	–	–	–	–
Total	100	100	100	100	100	100	100	100	100	100	100
Mean	**0.5**	**0.7**	**1.1**	**1.2**	**1.2**	**1.0**	**0.7**	**0.2**	**0.1**	**–**	**–**
Decayed (d) + filled (f)											
0	53	47	38	33	30	38	54	77	90	95	98
1	13	12	10	15	15	17	15	12	6	3	1
2	9	9	12	14	16	15	12	6	3	1	–
3	7	8	10	12	11	12	7	2	1	–	–
4	7	8	9	9	10	8	5	1	–	–	–
5	4	6	9	7	9	5	3	1	–	–	–
6	3	5	4	5	4	3	2	–	–	–	–
7	2	1	3	3	2	1	1	–	–	–	–
8	1	3	2	1	1	1	–	–	–	–	–
9	1	–	1	1	–	–	–	–	–	–	–
10	–	1	–	–	–	–	–	–	–	–	–
11 or more	–	–	–	–	–	–	–	–	–	–	–
Total	100	100	100	100	100	100	100	100	100	100	100
Mean	**1.6**	**1.9**	**2.3**	**2.2**	**2.2**	**1.7**	**1.2**	**0.4**	**0.1**	**0.1**	**–**
Base	671	717	772	811	891	983	989	971	991	1,042	967
Wales											
Decayed (d)											
0	52	46	47	38	42	55	71	83	93	99	99
1	12	16	21	25	20	21	17	8	5	1	1
2	11	15	8	13	13	10	7	6	1	–	–
3	6	7	11	11	12	9	3	2	1	–	–
4	6	5	5	6	8	2	2	1	–	–	–
5	4	3	2	4	4	1	1	–	–	–	–
6	3	3	1	2	1	1	–	–	–	–	–
7	1	2	1	1	–	–	–	–	–	–	–
8	1	–	1	–	–	–	–	–	–	–	–
9	1	1	1	–	–	–	–	–	–	–	–
10	2	–	–	–	–	–	–	–	–	–	–
11 or more	1	–	–	–	–	–	–	–	–	–	–
Total	100	100	100	100	100	100	100	100	100	100	100
Mean	**1.8**	**1.7**	**1.4**	**1.5**	**1.4**	**0.9**	**0.5**	**0.3**	**0.1**	**–**	**–**

Appendix Table 3 *continued*

Number of deciduous teeth	Age (years)										
	5	6	7	8	9	10	11	12	13	14	15
	%	%	%	%	%	%	%	%	%	%	%
Filled (f) **Wales** *continued*											
0	65	62	60	53	52	57	74	89	95	98	100
1	14	16	14	16	15	19	12	7	3	1	–
2	9	5	9	12	15	8	7	3	1	–	–
3	6	6	8	5	7	7	4	1	–	–	–
4	3	8	5	6	5	4	1	–	–	–	–
5	2	2	2	4	4	2	1	–	–	–	–
6	1	2	2	1	1	2	–	–	–	–	–
7	–	–	–	2	–	–	–	–	–	–	–
8 or more	–	–	–	1	1	–	–	–	–	–	–
Total	100	100	100	100	100	100	100	100	100	100	100
Mean	**0.8**	**1.0**	**1.0**	**1.3**	**1.2**	**1.0**	**0.5**	**0.2**	**0.1**	**–**	**–**
Decayed (d) + filled (f)											
0	34	32	31	20	22	35	58	75	90	98	99
1	14	14	17	15	13	17	15	12	5	1	1
2	12	13	11	15	16	12	11	7	2	1	–
3	10	8	13	16	15	16	6	3	1	–	–
4	11	11	7	10	12	8	5	1	1	–	–
5	6	8	7	10	10	5	1	1	–	–	–
6	4	3	6	6	5	4	3	–	–	–	–
7	2	4	3	4	3	2	–	–	–	–	–
8	2	3	2	3	2	–	–	–	–	–	–
9	2	1	1	–	–	–	–	–	–	–	–
10	2	–	1	–	–	–	–	–	–	–	–
11 or more	1	1	–	–	–	–	–	–	–	–	–
Total	100	100	100	100	100	100	100	100	100	100	100
Mean	**2.6**	**2.7**	**2.4**	**2.8**	**2.7**	**1.9**	**1.0**	**0.5**	**0.2**	**–**	**–**
Base	*190*	*211*	*225*	*213*	*262*	*249*	*272*	*258*	*281*	*264*	*279*
Scotland											
Decayed (d)											
0	34	38	35	30	40	55	69	87	94	99	99
1	13	14	16	21	24	22	15	9	4	1	1
2	13	16	16	17	16	13	9	3	2	–	–
3	10	8	13	13	9	5	3	1	1	–	–
4	7	8	9	6	5	4	1	1	–	–	–
5	7	6	5	5	2	1	1	–	–	–	–
6	4	2	2	5	1	–	–	–	–	–	–
7	3	3	2	2	–	–	–	–	–	–	–
8	1	2	1	1	–	–	–	–	–	–	–
9	3	1	1	–	–	–	–	–	–	–	–
10	2	1	–	–	–	–	–	–	–	–	–
11 or more	1	–	–	–	–	–	–	–	–	–	–
Total	100	100	100	100	100	100	100	100	100	100	100
Mean	**2.6**	**2.1**	**1.9**	**2.0**	**1.4**	**0.9**	**0.6**	**0.2**	**0.1**	**–**	**–**
Filled (f)											
0	74	59	57	51	55	63	80	89	97	99	99
1	10	15	15	17	17	19	11	6	3	1	1
2	7	8	9	10	11	9	5	3	–	1	–
3	4	7	7	9	6	5	2	1	1	–	–
4	3	5	6	6	5	3	1	–	–	–	–
5	2	4	3	4	2	1	1	–	–	–	–
6	–	3	1	1	1	1	–	–	–	–	–
7	–	–	1	1	–	–	–	–	–	–	–
8 or more	–	–	1	–	1	–	–	–	–	–	–
Total	100	100	100	100	100	100	100	100	100	100	100
Mean	**0.6**	**1.1**	**1.1**	**1.3**	**1.1**	**1.7**	**0.4**	**0.2**	**–**	**–**	**–**
Decayed (d) + filled (f)											
0	26	25	22	15	22	38	59	78	92	98	98
1	10	11	10	14	16	20	15	11	4	1	2
2	14	11	12	13	19	15	12	7	2	1	–
3	10	11	17	16	15	10	6	2	1	–	–
4	8	11	15	11	10	9	3	1	–	–	–
5	9	10	9	10	8	6	3	–	–	–	–
6	8	7	6	11	6	2	1	–	–	–	–
7	3	5	4	6	1	1	–	–	–	–	–
8	2	3	4	3	2	–	–	–	–	–	–
9	3	2	1	1	–	–	–	–	–	–	–
10	3	2	–	–	–	–	–	–	–	–	–
11 or more	1	1	–	–	–	–	–	–	–	–	–
Total	100	100	100	100	100	100	100	100	100	100	100
Mean	**3.2**	**3.2**	**3.0**	**3.3**	**2.5**	**1.6**	**0.9**	**0.4**	**0.1**	**–**	**–**
Base	*319*	*357*	*357*	*412*	*401*	*416*	*479*	*525*	*507*	*588*	*486*

Appendix Table 3 continued

Number of deciduous teeth	Age (years)										
	5	6	7	8	9	10	11	12	13	14	15
	%	%	%	%	%	%	%	%	%	%	%
	Northern Ireland										
Decayed (d)											
0	32	38	28	30	39	38	72	84	94	98	99
1	11	16	20	20	23	29	13	10	4	2	–
2	11	11	13	22	18	16	9	5	1	–	–
3	10	9	11	12	10	11	4	–	–	–	–
4	9	8	9	7	6	4	2	1	–	–	–
5	8	6	5	5	2	1	–	–	–	–	–
6	5	2	2	1	1	1	–	–	–	–	–
7	4	4	4	1	–	–	–	–	–	–	–
8	5	1	3	–	–	–	–	–	–	–	–
9	2	1	1	–	–	–	–	–	–	–	–
10	2	–	–	–	–	–	–	–	–	–	–
11 or more	1	–	–	–	–	–	–	–	–	–	–
Total	100	100	100	100	100	100	100	100	100	100	100
Mean	**3.0**	**2.2**	**2.5**	**1.8**	**1.4**	**1.2**	**0.5**	**0.3**	**0.1**	**–**	**–**
Filled (f)											
0	74	68	59	53	60	64	79	93	96	99	100
1	7	7	13	19	12	14	8	5	4	1	–
2	7	10	10	10	11	12	6	1	–	–	–
3	5	7	7	6	7	6	4	1	–	–	–
4	4	6	3	3	4	2	2	–	–	–	–
5	2	1	3	5	3	1	–	–	–	–	–
6	1	–	1	2	3	1	–	–	–	–	–
7	2	–	1	–	–	–	–	–	–	–	–
8 or more	1	–	–	–	–	–	–	–	–	–	–
Total	100	100	100	100	100	100	100	100	100	100	100
Mean	**0.7**	**0.8**	**1.1**	**1.2**	**1.0**	**0.8**	**0.4**	**0.1**	**–**	**–**	**–**
Decayed (d) + filled (f)											
0	26	25	16	16	22	27	58	80	92	97	99
1	8	10	10	11	14	18	15	10	5	3	–
2	11	11	12	20	20	21	12	5	2	–	1
3	7	13	16	16	15	13	6	2	–	–	–
4	11	17	14	10	14	12	5	2	–	–	–
5	8	9	9	16	7	5	3	–	–	–	–
6	9	4	8	5	5	3	–	–	–	–	–
7	6	6	6	3	2	1	–	–	–	–	–
8	7	1	3	2	–	–	–	–	–	–	–
9	4	1	2	–	–	–	–	–	–	–	–
10	1	–	–	–	–	–	–	–	–	–	–
11 or more	1	–	–	–	–	–	–	–	–	–	–
Total	100	100	100	100	100	100	100	100	100	100	100
Mean	**3.7**	**3.0**	**3.5**	**3.0**	**2.4**	**2.0**	**0.9**	**0.4**	**0.1**	**–**	**–**
Base	198	202	201	202	225	224	233	239	276	227	217

Appendix Table 4 Distribution of the number of permanent teeth which are decayed, missing or filled by age: United Kingdom and constituent countries

Number of permanent teeth	Age (years)										
	5	6	7	8	9	10	11	12	13	14	15
	%	%	%	%	%	%	%	%	%	%	%
United Kingdom											
Decayed (D)											
0	99	95	89	81	79	73	70	68	66	61	58
1	–	3	7	11	12	15	16	17	17	18	19
2	–	1	3	5	6	7	7	8	8	9	9
3	–	–	1	1	2	2	4	4	5	5	6
4	–	–	1	2	1	2	2	1	2	3	4
5	–	–	–	–	–	–	1	1	1	1	1
6	–	–	–	–	–	–	–	1	1	1	1
7	–	–	–	–	–	–	–	–	–	1	1
8	–	–	–	–	–	–	–	–	–	1	–
9	–	–	–	–	–	–	–	–	–	–	–
10	–	–	–	–	–	–	–	–	–	–	–
11 or more	–	–	–	–	–	–	–	–	–	–	–
Total	100	100	100	100	100	100	100	100	100	100	100
Mean	–	**0.1**	**0.2**	**0.3**	**0.4**	**0.5**	**0.6**	**0.6**	**0.7**	**0.9**	**1.0**
Missing (M)											
0	100	100	100	98	96	94	90	86	84	81	76
1	–	–	–	1	1	2	4	6	6	8	8
2	–	–	–	1	1	2	3	4	5	5	8
3	–	–	–	–	–	–	1	1	1	2	3
4	–	–	–	–	1	2	2	3	4	4	5
5	–	–	–	–	–	–	–	–	–	–	–
6	–	–	–	–	–	–	–	–	–	–	–
7	–	–	–	–	–	–	–	–	–	–	–
8 or more	–	–	–	–	–	–	–	–	–	–	–
Total	100	100	100	100	100	100	100	100	100	100	100
Mean	–	–	–	–	**0.1**	**0.1**	**0.2**	**0.3**	**0.4**	**0.4**	**0.6**
Filled (F)											
0	100	97	89	75	62	53	43	31	28	20	15
1	–	2	5	10	13	14	14	16	11	9	7
2	–	1	4	8	11	12	14	15	13	11	10
3	–	–	1	3	7	9	11	12	12	13	12
4	–	–	1	4	7	10	13	15	14	14	14
5	–	–	–	–	–	1	1	4	7	8	10
6	–	–	–	–	–	–	1	3	5	7	7
7	–	–	–	–	–	–	1	2	3	5	7
8	–	–	–	–	–	–	–	1	3	5	6
9	–	–	–	–	–	–	–	–	2	3	4
10	–	–	–	–	–	–	–	–	–	2	2
11 or more	–	–	–	–	–	–	–	–	–	1	2
Total	100	100	100	100	100	100	100	100	100	100	100
Mean	–	–	**0.2**	**0.5**	**0.8**	**1.2**	**1.6**	**2.1**	**2.8**	**3.6**	**4.4**
Base	*804*	*863*	*921*	*968*	*1,061*	*1,152*	*1,177*	*1,165*	*1,192*	*1,248*	*1,156*
England and Wales											
Decayed (D)											
0	99	96	90	83	81	75	72	70	68	63	60
1	–	3	6	10	11	14	15	17	16	18	19
2	–	1	3	4	5	7	6	7	8	9	9
3	–	–	1	1	2	2	4	3	4	4	6
4	–	–	–	1	1	1	2	1	1	3	4
5	–	–	–	–	–	–	1	1	1	1	1
6	–	–	–	–	–	–	–	1	1	1	1
7	–	–	–	–	–	–	–	–	–	–	–
8	–	–	–	–	–	–	–	–	–	1	–
9	–	–	–	–	–	–	–	–	–	–	–
10	–	–	–	–	–	–	–	–	–	–	–
11 or more	–	–	–	–	–	–	–	–	–	–	–
Total	100	100	100	100	100	100	100	100	100	100	100
Mean	–	**0.1**	**0.2**	**0.3**	**0.3**	**0.4**	**0.5**	**0.6**	**0.7**	**0.8**	**0.9**
Missing (M)											
0	100	100	100	98	97	95	92	88	86	84	78
1	–	–	–	1	1	2	4	5	5	8	7
2	–	–	–	1	1	1	2	3	4	4	7
3	–	–	–	–	–	–	–	–	1	1	2
4	–	–	–	–	1	2	2	3	3	3	5
5	–	–	–	–	–	–	–	–	–	–	–
6	–	–	–	–	–	–	–	–	–	–	–
7	–	–	–	–	–	–	–	–	–	–	–
8 or more	–	–	–	–	–	–	–	–	–	–	–
Total	100	100	100	100	100	100	100	100	100	100	100
Mean	–	–	–	–	**0.1**	**0.1**	**0.2**	**0.3**	**0.3**	**0.3**	**0.5**

Number of permanent teeth	Age (years)										
	5	6	7	8	9	10	11	12	13	14	15
	%	%	%	%	%	%	%	%	%	%	%

England and Wales *continued*

Filled (F)

	5	6	7	8	9	10	11	12	13	14	15
0	100	97	90	77	64	54	44	32	29	21	15
1	–	2	5	10	13	14	15	17	12	10	8
2	–	–	4	7	11	12	14	15	13	11	11
3	–	–	1	2	6	9	11	11	12	13	12
4	–	–	1	3	6	10	13	15	14	14	14
5	–	–	–	–	–	1	1	4	7	8	10
6	–	–	–	–	–	–	1	3	5	7	7
7	–	–	–	–	–	–	1	2	3	5	7
8	–	–	–	–	–	–	–	1	2	5	6
9	–	–	–	–	–	–	–	–	1	2	4
10	–	–	–	–	–	–	–	–	–	2	2
11 or more	–	–	–	–	–	–	–	–	–	1	2
Total	100	100	100	100	100	100	100	100	100	100	100
Mean	**–**	**–**	**0.2**	**0.4**	**0.8**	**1.1**	**1.5**	**2.1**	**2.7**	**3.5**	**4.2**
Base	*719*	*770*	*829*	*865*	*957*	*1,046*	*1,058*	*1,036*	*1,062*	*1,109*	*1,038*

England

Decayed (D)

	5	6	7	8	9	10	11	12	13	14	15
0	99	96	90	83	81	75	72	70	69	63	60
1	–	3	6	10	11	15	15	17	16	18	19
2	–	1	3	4	5	7	6	7	7	8	9
3	–	–	1	1	2	2	4	3	4	4	5
4	–	–	–	1	1	1	2	1	1	3	4
5	–	–	–	–	–	–	1	1	1	1	1
6	–	–	–	–	–	–	–	1	1	1	1
7	–	–	–	–	–	–	–	–	–	–	–
8	–	–	–	–	–	–	–	–	–	–	–
9	–	–	–	–	–	–	–	–	–	–	–
10	–	–	–	–	–	–	–	–	–	–	–
11 or more	–	–	–	–	–	–	–	–	–	–	–
Total	100	100	100	100	100	100	100	100	100	100	100
Mean	**–**	**0.1**	**0.2**	**0.3**	**0.3**	**0.4**	**0.5**	**0.6**	**0.6**	**0.8**	**0.9**

Missing (M)

	5	6	7	8	9	10	11	12	13	14	15
0	100	100	100	98	97	95	92	88	86	84	79
1	–	–	–	1	1	2	3	5	5	7	7
2	–	–	–	1	1	1	2	3	4	4	7
3	–	–	–	–	–	–	–	–	1	1	2
4	–	–	–	–	1	2	2	3	3	3	5
5	–	–	–	–	–	–	–	–	–	–	–
6	–	–	–	–	–	–	–	–	–	–	–
7	–	–	–	–	–	–	–	–	–	–	–
8 or more	–	–	–	–	–	–	–	–	–	–	–
Total	100	100	100	100	100	100	100	100	100	100	100
Mean	**–**	**–**	**–**	**–**	**0.1**	**0.1**	**0.2**	**0.3**	**0.3**	**0.3**	**0.5**

Filled (F)

	5	6	7	8	9	10	11	12	13	14	15
0	100	97	90	78	64	55	44	32	29	21	15
1	–	2	5	10	13	14	15	17	12	10	8
2	–	–	4	7	11	11	14	15	13	11	11
3	–	–	1	2	6	9	11	11	13	13	12
4	–	–	1	3	6	10	13	15	14	14	14
5	–	–	–	–	–	1	1	4	7	8	10
6	–	–	–	–	–	–	1	2	5	7	7
7	–	–	–	–	–	–	1	2	3	5	7
8	–	–	–	–	–	–	–	1	2	5	6
9	–	–	–	–	–	–	–	–	1	2	4
10	–	–	–	–	–	–	–	–	–	2	2
11 or more	–	–	–	–	–	–	–	–	–	1	2
Total	100	100	100	100	100	100	100	100	100	100	100
Mean	**–**	**–**	**0.2**	**0.4**	**0.8**	**1.1**	**1.5**	**2.0**	**2.7**	**3.5**	**4.2**
Base	*671*	*717*	*772*	*811*	*891*	*983*	*989*	*971*	*991*	*1,042*	*967*

Wales

Decayed (D)

	5	6	7	8	9	10	11	12	13	14	15
0	99	95	92	83	79	79	63	67	60	58	54
1	1	4	5	10	11	12	19	14	18	18	18
2	–	1	3	6	6	5	7	11	10	9	10
3	–	–	–	1	2	1	6	4	2	6	8
4	–	–	–	–	2	2	3	2	2	3	4
5	–	–	–	–	–	1	1	1	4	2	2
6	–	–	–	–	–	–	1	–	1	–	3
7	–	–	–	–	–	–	–	–	1	1	–
8	–	–	–	–	–	–	–	–	–	1	–
9	–	–	–	–	–	–	–	–	–	–	–
10	–	–	–	–	–	–	–	–	–	1	–
11 or more	–	–	–	–	–	–	–	–	–	–	–
Total	100	100	100	100	100	100	100	100	100	100	100
Mean	**–**	**0.1**	**0.1**	**0.3**	**0.4**	**0.4**	**0.8**	**0.7**	**0.9**	**1.1**	**1.2**

Appendix Table 4 *continued*

Number of permanent teeth	Age (years)										
	5	6	7	8	9	10	11	12	13	14	15
	%	%	%	%	%	%	%	%	%	%	%
Wales *continued*											
Missing (M)											
0	100	100	100	98	96	92	87	83	76	76	66
1	–	–	–	–	2	3	6	6	10	8	13
2	–	–	–	1	2	3	3	6	9	7	10
3	–	–	–	–	–	–	1	2	1	5	2
4	–	–	–	–	–	1	3	3	3	4	8
5	–	–	–	–	–	–	–	–	–	–	–
6	–	–	–	–	–	–	–	–	1	–	1
7	–	–	–	–	–	–	–	–	–	–	–
8 or more	–	–	–	–	–	–	–	–	–	–	–
Total	100	100	100	100	100	100	100	100	100	100	100
Mean	–	–	–	–	**0.1**	**0.2**	**0.3**	**0.3**	**0.5**	**0.5**	**0.8**
Filled (F)											
0	99	98	91	71	60	47	42	28	26	17	13
1	1	1	5	10	16	18	15	15	10	8	8
2	–	1	4	9	12	16	15	15	14	11	11
3	–	–	–	5	7	10	11	15	10	13	9
4	–	–	–	5	6	9	11	12	14	18	13
5	–	–	–	–	–	–	3	6	9	7	9
6	–	–	–	–	–	–	2	4	6	6	7
7	–	–	–	–	–	–	–	2	4	6	9
8	–	–	–	–	–	–	–	1	3	6	8
9	–	–	–	–	–	–	–	–	1	3	4
10	–	–	–	–	–	–	–	1	1	1	3
11 or more	–	–	–	–	–	–	–	–	1	1	1
Total	100	100	100	100	100	100	100	100	100	100	100
Mean	–	–	**0.2**	**0.6**	**0.8**	**1.2**	**1.6**	**2.3**	**3.0**	**4.0**	**4.8**
Base	*190*	*211*	*225*	*213*	*262*	*249*	*272*	*258*	*281*	*264*	*279*
Scotland											
Decayed (D)											
0	98	93	76	68	65	60	62	59	49	48	45
1	1	4	11	17	15	21	18	17	17	19	21
2	1	2	7	7	10	10	8	12	13	10	11
3	–	–	3	4	6	4	6	4	10	7	8
4	–	1	2	4	3	4	4	3	4	5	6
5	–	–	–	–	–	–	–	2	2	4	3
6	–	–	–	–	–	–	1	1	1	2	3
7	–	–	–	–	–	–	–	–	1	1	1
8	–	–	–	–	–	–	–	1	1	1	1
9	–	–	–	–	–	–	–	–	–	1	1
10	–	–	–	–	–	–	–	–	1	1	–
11 or more	–	–	–	–	–	–	–	–	–	–	1
Total	100	100	100	100	100	100	100	100	100	100	100
Mean	–	**0.1**	**0.4**	**0.6**	**0.7**	**0.8**	**0.9**	**1.1**	**1.3**	**1.5**	**1.5**
Missing (M)											
0	100	100	99	96	91	85	82	75	69	61	56
1	–	–	1	2	4	6	6	9	10	14	13
2	–	–	1	1	3	6	7	9	10	9	12
3	–	–	–	–	–	–	1	2	3	4	7
4	–	–	–	1	1	2	3	5	7	9	10
5	–	–	–	–	–	–	–	–	–	2	1
6	–	–	–	–	–	–	–	–	–	–	1
7	–	–	–	–	–	–	–	–	–	–	1
8 or more	–	–	–	–	–	–	–	–	–	–	–
Total	100	100	100	100	100	100	100	100	100	100	100
Mean	–	–	–	**0.1**	**0.2**	**0.3**	**0.4**	**0.6**	**0.7**	**1.0**	**1.1**
Filled (F)											
0	100	96	81	61	51	39	29	23	18	17	10
1	–	3	10	13	13	16	12	14	8	8	6
2	–	1	6	15	13	15	16	13	13	11	9
3	–	1	2	6	8	13	14	14	12	9	9
4	–	–	1	5	12	13	18	17	14	13	9
5	–	–	–	–	–	2	4	6	9	10	11
6	–	–	–	–	1	1	3	4	7	7	8
7	–	–	–	–	–	–	1	2	5	6	6
8	–	–	–	–	–	–	2	3	4	5	9
9	–	–	–	–	–	–	–	1	4	5	6
10	–	–	–	–	–	–	–	1	2	3	6
11 or more	–	–	–	–	–	–	–	–	1	2	3
Total	100	100	100	100	100	100	100	100	100	100	100
Mean	–	**0.1**	**0.3**	**0.8**	**1.2**	**1.6**	**2.3**	**2.9**	**3.8**	**4.3**	**5.8**
Base	*319*	*357*	*357*	*412*	*401*	*416*	*479*	*525*	*507*	*588*	*486*

Appendix Table 4 *continued*

Number of permanent teeth	Age (years)										
	5	6	7	8	9	10	11	12	13	14	15
	%	%	%	%	%	%	%	%	%	%	%
	Northern Ireland										
Decayed (D)											
0	96	90	65	62	56	52	46	43	36	45	36
1	2	5	18	19	17	16	22	19	24	20	20
2	1	3	7	10	13	16	12	12	15	11	11
3	1	–	5	5	8	8	8	12	9	7	8
4	–	1	4	3	3	6	5	6	6	7	7
5	–	–	–	–	2	–	3	3	4	1	3
6	–	–	–	–	–	–	2	3	1	3	6
7	–	–	–	–	–	–	–	2	2	2	4
8	–	–	–	–	–	–	–	–	2	1	2
9	–	–	–	–	–	–	–	–	–	1	1
10	–	–	–	–	–	–	1	–	–	1	–
11 or more	–	–	–	–	–	–	–	–	–	1	–
Total	100	100	100	100	100	100	100	100	100	100	100
Mean	**0.1**	**0.2**	**0.7**	**0.7**	**0.9**	**1.1**	**1.3**	**1.5**	**1.8**	**1.7**	**2.1**
Missing (M)											
0	100	100	98	93	89	85	74	69	59	60	47
1	–	–	2	3	4	5	11	10	14	15	18
2	–	–	–	2	4	6	8	7	15	9	16
3	–	–	–	–	1	1	2	6	3	4	7
4	–	–	–	1	2	3	5	8	8	8	9
5	–	–	–	–	–	–	–	–	1	1	1
6	–	–	–	–	–	–	–	–	–	2	1
7	–	–	–	–	–	–	–	–	–	–	–
8 or more	–	–	–	–	–	–	–	–	–	–	–
Total	100	100	100	100	100	100	100	100	100	100	100
Mean	**–**	**–**	**–**	**0.1**	**0.2**	**0.3**	**0.6**	**0.7**	**0.9**	**1.0**	**1.3**
Filled (F)											
0	99	92	82	61	46	41	32	34	25	21	17
1	1	4	9	9	12	11	15	8	8	6	4
2	–	2	4	9	14	15	16	15	12	7	6
3	–	1	1	8	12	9	9	9	11	12	11
4	–	–	4	11	14	21	19	14	13	13	8
5	–	–	–	–	1	2	3	6	8	5	5
6	–	–	–	–	–	–	3	4	5	4	6
7	–	–	–	–	–	1	1	5	7	4	10
8	–	–	–	–	–	–	–	–	3	6	7
9	–	–	–	–	–	–	–	1	1	5	6
10	–	–	–	–	–	–	–	2	2	4	3
11 or more	–	–	–	–	–	–	1	1	1	4	5
Total	100	100	100	100	100	100	100	100	100	100	100
Mean	**–**	**0.1**	**0.4**	**1.0**	**1.4**	**1.7**	**2.1**	**2.6**	**3.6**	**5.1**	**5.8**
Base	198	202	201	202	225	224	233	239	276	227	217

Appendix Table 5 Distribution of the number of permanent teeth with decay experience, by age: United Kingdom and constituent countries

Number of permanent teeth that are, or have been decayed	Age (years)										
	5	6	7	8	9	10	11	12	13	14	15
	%	%	%	%	%	%	%	%	%	%	%
United Kingdom											
0	99	92	79	62	49	37	28	19	17	11	7
1	–	5	9	14	14	15	13	12	9	7	4
2	–	2	7	10	13	14	13	14	10	9	7
3	–	–	3	5	8	11	13	11	11	10	9
4	–	1	2	8	13	19	22	21	19	15	14
5	–	–	–	–	1	2	5	7	10	10	11
6	–	–	–	–	–	1	2	5	8	8	8
7	–	–	–	–	–	–	1	3	5	7	9
8	–	–	–	–	–	–	1	3	4	8	9
9	–	–	–	–	–	–	1	1	2	5	6
10	–	–	–	–	–	–	–	–	1	3	4
11	–	–	–	–	–	–	–	–	1	2	3
12	–	–	–	–	–	–	–	–	1	1	3
13	–	–	–	–	–	–	–	–	1	1	2
14	–	–	–	–	–	–	–	–	1	1	1
15	–	–	–	–	–	–	–	–	–	–	1
16	–	–	–	–	–	–	–	–	–	–	1
17	–	–	–	–	–	–	–	–	–	–	1
18	–	–	–	–	–	–	–	–	–	–	–
19	–	–	–	–	–	–	–	–	–	–	–
20 or more	–	–	–	–	–	–	–	–	–	–	–
Total	100	100	100	100	100	100	100	100	100	100	100
Base	*804*	*863*	*921*	*968*	*1,061*	*1,152*	*1,177*	*1,165*	*1,192*	*1,248*	*1,156*
England and Wales											
0	99	93	81	65	52	39	30	21	19	12	8
1	–	5	8	14	15	16	14	13	9	8	5
2	–	1	6	10	13	14	13	15	10	9	7
3	–	–	2	4	8	10	13	12	11	10	10
4	–	1	2	7	12	18	21	21	19	16	15
5	–	–	–	–	1	2	4	7	10	10	11
6	–	–	–	–	–	1	2	5	7	8	8
7	–	–	–	–	–	–	1	3	5	7	9
8	–	–	–	–	–	–	1	3	3	8	9
9	–	–	–	–	–	–	–	1	2	4	5
10	–	–	–	–	–	–	–	–	1	3	4
11	–	–	–	–	–	–	–	–	1	2	2
12	–	–	–	–	–	–	–	–	1	1	3
13	–	–	–	–	–	–	–	–	–	1	2
14	–	–	–	–	–	–	–	–	1	1	1
15	–	–	–	–	–	–	–	–	–	–	1
16	–	–	–	–	–	–	–	–	–	–	–
17	–	–	–	–	–	–	–	–	–	–	1
18	–	–	–	–	–	–	–	–	–	–	–
19	–	–	–	–	–	–	–	–	–	–	–
20 or more	–	–	–	–	–	–	–	–	–	–	–
Total	100	100	100	100	100	100	100	100	100	100	100
Base	*719*	*770*	*829*	*865*	*957*	*1,046*	*1,058*	*1,036*	*1,062*	*1,109*	*1,038*
England											
0	99	93	81	65	52	39	31	21	19	13	8
1	–	5	8	14	15	16	14	13	9	8	5
2	–	1	6	10	12	14	13	15	10	9	7
3	–	–	2	4	8	10	12	11	11	10	10
4	–	1	2	7	12	18	21	20	19	15	15
5	–	–	–	–	1	2	4	7	10	10	11
6	–	–	–	–	–	1	2	5	7	8	8
7	–	–	–	–	–	–	1	3	5	7	9
8	–	–	–	–	–	–	1	3	3	8	9
9	–	–	–	–	–	–	–	1	2	4	5
10	–	–	–	–	–	–	–	–	1	3	4
11	–	–	–	–	–	–	–	–	1	2	2
12	–	–	–	–	–	–	–	–	1	1	3
13	–	–	–	–	–	–	–	–	–	1	2
14	–	–	–	–	–	–	–	–	1	1	1
15	–	–	–	–	–	–	–	–	–	–	1
16	–	–	–	–	–	–	–	–	–	–	–
17	–	–	–	–	–	–	–	–	–	–	1
18	–	–	–	–	–	–	–	–	–	–	–
19	–	–	–	–	–	–	–	–	–	–	–
20 or more	–	–	–	–	–	–	–	–	–	–	–
Total	100	100	100	100	100	100	100	100	100	100	100
Base	*671*	*717*	*772*	*811*	*891*	*983*	*989*	*971*	*991*	*1,042*	*967*

Appendix Table 5 *continued*

Number of permanent teeth that are, or have been decayed	Age (years)										
	5	6	7	8	9	10	11	12	13	14	15
	%	%	%	%	%	%	%	%	%	%	%
Wales											
0	99	94	84	60	47	35	22	17	14	6	6
1	–	3	9	14	15	14	14	7	7	4	2
2	1	2	4	9	18	22	13	12	10	8	6
3	–	–	1	9	9	9	16	14	8	8	6
4	–	–	2	8	11	16	21	26	20	23	14
5	–	–	–	–	–	1	7	9	11	8	11
6	–	–	–	–	–	1	4	6	8	6	7
7	–	–	–	–	–	–	1	3	6	8	10
8	–	–	–	–	–	1	1	2	5	10	9
9	–	–	–	–	–	–	–	2	4	5	8
10	–	–	–	–	–	–	–	1	3	4	5
11	–	–	–	–	–	–	–	–	2	2	4
12	–	–	–	–	–	–	–	1	–	3	2
13	–	–	–	–	–	–	1	–	–	–	1
14	–	–	–	–	–	–	–	–	–	1	2
15	–	–	–	–	–	–	–	–	1	–	2
16	–	–	–	–	–	–	–	–	1	–	1
17	–	–	–	–	–	–	–	–	–	1	1
18	–	–	–	–	–	–	–	–	–	1	1
19	–	–	–	–	–	–	–	–	–	–	1
20 or more	–	–	–	–	–	–	–	–	–	–	–
Total	100	100	100	100	100	100	100	100	100	100	100
Base	*190*	*211*	*225*	*213*	*262*	*249*	*272*	*258*	*281*	*264*	*279*
Scotland											
0	98	89	63	40	30	21	12	10	6	5	2
1	1	7	14	16	14	13	9	8	3	2	2
2	1	3	10	15	15	12	12	9	5	7	4
3	–	1	6	13	11	14	15	9	7	7	2
4	–	1	6	16	24	27	29	26	18	13	7
5	–	–	–	1	3	6	8	11	13	11	10
6	–	–	–	–	1	3	5	8	10	11	10
7	–	–	–	–	–	1	3	5	8	8	7
8	–	–	–	–	–	1	2	5	11	7	12
9	–	–	–	–	–	–	1	3	4	6	7
10	–	–	–	–	–	–	1	2	4	5	7
11	–	–	–	–	–	–	1	1	4	3	6
12	–	–	–	–	–	–	1	2	2	4	5
13	–	–	–	–	–	–	1	–	2	3	4
14	–	–	–	–	–	–	–	1	–	2	3
15	–	–	–	–	–	–	–	1	2	2	3
16	–	–	–	–	–	–	–	–	1	1	3
17	–	–	–	–	–	–	–	1	1	1	1
18	–	–	–	–	–	–	–	–	–	1	1
19	–	–	–	–	–	–	–	–	–	–	1
20 or more	–	–	–	–	–	–	–	–	–	1	1
Total	100	100	100	100	100	100	100	100	100	100	100
Base	*319*	*357*	*357*	*412*	*401*	*416*	*479*	*525*	*507*	*588*	*486*
Northern Ireland											
0	96	83	55	32	21	14	9	6	3	4	–
1	3	7	16	16	11	7	9	5	4	2	2
2	1	6	10	15	13	15	11	7	5	3	2
3	1	1	7	10	16	14	9	11	7	11	5
4	–	2	11	24	29	35	35	26	15	15	7
5	–	–	–	2	6	7	9	13	15	7	5
6	–	–	–	–	4	3	5	10	11	6	8
7	–	–	–	–	–	2	3	8	11	5	8
8	–	–	–	–	–	2	3	4	8	11	8
9	–	–	–	–	–	–	3	3	5	5	13
10	–	–	–	–	–	–	1	1	3	5	11
11	–	–	–	–	–	–	2	3	4	6	7
12	–	–	–	–	–	–	–	–	2	4	3
13	–	–	–	–	–	–	–	3	1	3	4
14	–	–	–	–	–	–	–	1	–	4	3
15	–	–	–	–	–	–	–	–	2	2	4
16	–	–	–	–	–	–	–	–	1	1	4
17	–	–	–	–	–	–	–	–	1	2	3
18	–	–	–	–	–	–	–	–	–	1	–
19	–	–	–	–	–	–	–	–	1	–	1
20 or more	–	–	–	–	–	–	–	–	–	1	1
Total	100	100	100	100	100	100	100	100	100	100	100
Base	*198*	*202*	*201*	*202*	*225*	*224*	*233*	*239*	*276*	*227*	*217*

Appendix Table 6 Comparison of the condition of deciduous and permanent teeth among children in England and Wales, 1973 and 1983

Age (years)	Deciduous teeth						Permanent teeth							
	Decayed (d)		Filled (f)		Decayed or filled (df)		Decayed (D)		Missing (M)		Filled (F)		Decayed missing or filled (DMF)	
	1973	1983	1973	1983	1973	1983	1973	1983	1973	1983	1973	1983	1973	1983
Average number of teeth which are...														
5	2.6	1.1	0.7	0.5	3.3	1.6	0.0	0.0	0.0	0.0	0.0	0.0	0.0	0.0
6	2.5	1.2	1.0	0.7	3.6	1.9	0.2	0.1	0.0	0.0	0.1	0.0	0.3	0.1
7	2.3	1.2	1.1	1.1	3.4	2.3	0.5	0.2	0.0	0.0	0.3	0.2	0.8	0.3
8	2.0	1.1	1.2	1.2	3.3	2.2	0.8	0.3	0.1	0.0	0.9	0.4	1.7	0.7
9	1.6	1.0	1.1	1.2	2.8	2.2	0.8	0.3	0.1	0.1	1.2	0.8	2.2	1.2
10	1.2	0.7	0.7	1.0	1.9	1.7	1.0	0.4	0.3	0.1	1.7	1.1	3.0	1.7
11	0.6	0.5	0.4	0.7	1.0	1.2	1.3	0.5	0.4	0.2	2.2	1.5	3.9	2.2
12	0.2	0.2	0.2	0.2	0.4	0.4	1.4	0.6	0.5	0.3	2.9	2.1	4.8	2.9
13	0.1	0.1	0.0	0.1	0.2	0.2	1.6	0.7	0.6	0.3	3.8	2.7	6.1	3.7
14	0.0	0.0	0.0	0.0	0.0	0.1	1.9	0.8	0.8	0.3	4.8	3.5	7.4	4.7
15	0.0	0.0	0.0	0.0	0.0	0.0	1.6	0.9	0.8	0.5	6.0	4.2	8.4	5.6
Proportion of children with some teeth which are...														
5	63%	38%	26%	23%	71%	48%	3%	1%	–	–	–	–	3%	1%
6	68%	43%	38%	30%	79%	54%	12%	4%	–	–	5%	3%	16%	7%
7	68%	45%	42%	40%	83%	62%	27%	10%	1%	–	17%	10%	39%	19%
8	72%	47%	45%	47%	85%	68%	40%	17%	4%	2%	37%	23%	65%	35%
9	66%	49%	44%	50%	81%	71%	42%	19%	8%	3%	50%	36%	74%	48%
10	51%	39%	33%	43%	63%	62%	46%	25%	13%	5%	61%	46%	85%	61%
11	32%	28%	21%	32%	43%	46%	53%	28%	18%	8%	66%	56%	90%	70%
12	15%	14%	10%	13%	21%	23%	54%	30%	23%	12%	75%	68%	93%	79%
13	7%	5%	4%	6%	10%	10%	58%	32%	28%	14%	77%	71%	95%	81%
14	2%	2%	1%	3%	3%	5%	61%	37%	31%	16%	81%	79%	96%	88%
15	1%	1%	1%	1%	1%	2%	57%	40%	33%	22%	88%	85%	97%	92%

Appendix F The documents

S1189

Office of Population Censuses and Surveys

St Catherines House 10 Kingsway London WC2B 6JP

Telephone 01-242 0262 ext 2276

Serial No:
F 3-9

Date:
10-15

Dear Parent,

We sent you a letter a little while ago about a survey of children's dental health that we are carrying out throughout the country for the United Kingdom Health Departments. The survey will show us how much dental decay children have these days and what kind of dental treatment is provided.

A sample of school children has been selected to be examined by the dentist at school and this examination will tell us about the dental condition of children's teeth. However there are some other things which would complete the dental picture which only you could tell us about, things about visiting the dentist, cleaning teeth and so on.

I am writing to ask you if you would help us by answering the questions on this form and returning it to us in the enclosed envelope.

The information you give will be treated in strict confidence and used for statistical purposes only. Nothing that would identify you will be passed on by us to any other government department or organization.

I do hope you will feel able to help us in this way, in which case I thank you in advance for your co-operation.

Yours sincerely

Jean E. Todd.

Jean E Todd
Chief Social Survey Officer

HOW TO FILL IN THE FORM

1. Most questions on the following pages can be answered simply by putting a tick in the box next to the answer that applies to you.

   Example

   Yes ☐ 1

   No ☐ 2

   Sometimes you are asked to answer in your own words.

2. When the answer is a number, please fill it in as figures (not words) on the line provided.

3. Usually after answering each question you go on to the next one unless a box you have ticked has an arrow next to it with an instruction to go to another question.

   Example

   Yes ☐ 1 ⟶ GO TO Q4

   No ☐ 2

4. If you cannot remember, do not know, or are unable to answer, a particular question please write that in.

5. If you have more than one child please answer the questions in relation to the child whose name is printed on the label on page 1.

6. Teenage children may wish to fill in questions 1 to 34 themselves, if so they should tick the box at question 35. Would you please complete questions 36 to 44.

7. When you have finished, please post the questionnaire to us as soon as possible in the reply paid envelope provided, even if you were not able to answer all of it.

The names and addresses of people who co-operate in surveys are held in strict confidence and not passed on to any other Government department or to members of the public or press.

We are most grateful for your help and co-operation.

2

1. Has your child ever been to the dentist's surgery, either for treatment or just to get used to going?

   Yes [1] → Go to Q2
   No [2] → Go to Q14

   F 16

2. Thinking about the first time that your child ever went to the dentist. How old was he/she then? .... years old

   17 – 18

3. Why did he/she go the first time? Was it because ....   TICK ONE

   He/she was having trouble with his/her teeth? [1]
   You had a note from the school dentist? [2]
   He/she went for a check up? [3]
   He/she went just to get used to going to a dentist? [4]
   For some other reason (please tick and say what below) [5]

   19

4. Has your child ever had any dental treatment of any kind?

   Yes [1] → Go to Q5
   No [2] → Go to Q6

   20

5. What kind of treatment has your child had over the whole of his/her life so far?

   PLEASE TICK ALL THAT APPLY

   Teeth filled [1]
   Teeth taken out [2]
   A general anaesthetic when having a tooth taken out [3]
   Treatment to stop teeth decaying or going bad eg by painting and/or sealing the teeth [4]
   Other treatment (please tick and say what below) [5]

   21 – 25 (MC = 5)

3

---

6. Has your child been to the dentist ......   TICK ONE

   in the last 6 months? [1]
   longer ago but within the last year? [2]
   longer ago but within the last 2 years? [3]
   longer ago than 2 years? [4]

   F 26

7. Last time your child went to the dentist was it for just one visit or was it for more than one visit?

   One visit [1]
   More than one visit [2]

   27

8. Why did your child go to the dentist last time? (If he/she went for more than one visit last time, why did he/she go for the first visit?) Was it because ....   TICK ONE

   He/she was having trouble with his/her teeth? [1]
   You had a note from the school dentist? [2]
   He/she went for a check up? [3]
   For some other reason (please tick and say what below) [4]

   28

9. The last time your child went to the dentist, either for one visit or for several visits, did he/she have any treatment of any kind?

   Yes [1] → Go to Q10
   No [2] → Go to Q11

   29

10. What kind of treatment did he/she have?

    PLEASE TICK ALL THAT APPLY

    Teeth filled [1]
    Teeth taken out [2]
    Treatment to stop teeth decaying or going bad eg by painting and/or sealing the teeth [3]
    Other treatment (please tick and say what below) [4]

    F 30 – 33 (MC = 4)

4

142

11. Most treatment for children is free under the National Health Service, but sometimes it is done privately and has to be paid for.

Has your child ever had any treatment that you had to pay for?

Yes [1] → Go to Q12
No [2] → Go to Q13

34

12. What treatment did your child have that you had to pay for?

PLEASE TICK ALL THAT APPLY

Teeth filled [1]
Teeth taken out [2]
Treatment to stop teeth decaying or going bad eg by painting and/or sealing the teeth [3]
Other treatment (please tick and say what below) [4]

35 – 38
(MC = 4)

13. There are two main dental services for children, the National Health Service and the School Dental Service. Under which of these dental services has your child had dental treatment so far?

TICK ONE

National Health Service only [1]
School Dental Service only [2]
Both services [3]
Neither [4]

39

14. Has your child ever brought a note home from school asking if the school dentist can examine his/her teeth?

Yes [1]
No [2]

40

15. Has your child ever brought a note home from school, after the school dentist has examined him/her, to say that he/she should visit a dentist for treatment?

Yes [1]
No [2]

41

5

16. Do you think any of your child's teeth are decayed at the moment?

Yes [1]
No [2]

42

17. If your child had a bad back tooth and it was not a baby (milk) tooth but a second (permanent) tooth, would you rather it was filled or would you rather it was taken out?

Filled [1]
Taken out [2]

43

18. If your child had a bad front tooth and it was not a baby (milk) tooth but a second (permanent) tooth, would you rather it was filled or would you rather it was taken out?

Filled [1]
Taken out [2]

44

19. What do you think makes teeth decay (or go bad)? (PLEASE WRITE IN BELOW)

45 – 56
(MC = 6)

20. What do you think can be done to stop teeth decaying (or going bad)? (PLEASE WRITE IN BELOW)

57 – 68
(MC = 6)

6

143

PLEASE DO NOT WRITE IN THIS COLUMN

21. Most of the trouble that children have with their teeth is because of decay, but some children have other dental problems.

Has your child ever had a fall or some other accident that damaged any of his/her teeth?

Yes	1	→ Go to Q22	F 69
No	2	→ Go to Q25	

22. What was this damage?

PLEASE TICK ALL THAT APPLY

Teeth chipped, cracked, broken	1	
Teeth knocked loose	2	70 - 72 (MC = 3)
Teeth knocked out	3	

23. Was this damage to baby (milk) teeth, to second (permanent) teeth or to both?

TICK ONE

Baby teeth	1	
Second teeth	2	73
Both	3	

24. Did your child have to have any teeth taken out at the dentist because of this accident?

Yes	1	74
No	2	

25. Some children's teeth don't have enough room to grow and become crooked or protruding.

At this stage of growing up, are any of your child's teeth crooked at all, or not?

Yes	1	75
No	2	

26. At this stage of growing up, are any of your child's teeth protruding or sticking out?

Yes	1	76
No	2	79 - 80 = 06 END F

PLEASE DO NOT WRITE IN THIS COLUMN

27. Is your child having, or has your child ever had, treatment for crooked or protruding teeth?

Yes, having treatment now	1	→ Go to Q29	G
Yes, had treatment in the past	2	→ Go to Q28	10
No, no treatment	3	→ Go to Q28	

28. At the moment, do you think your child's teeth are alright as they are or would you prefer him/her to have them straightened?

Alright as they are	1	11
Prefer them to be straightened	2	

29. Does your child brush his/her teeth at all (or have them brushed for him/her)?

Yes	1	→ Go to Q30	12
No	2	→ Go to Q33	

30. Who usually brushes your child's teeth?

TICK ONE

Your child	1	
A parent	2	13
Parent and child together	3	
Other (please tick and write in below)	4	

31. How often does your child usually brush his/her teeth (or have them brushed for him/her)?

TICK ONE

More than 3 times a day	1	
3 times a day	2	
Twice a day	3	14
Once a day	4	
Less than once a day	5	

32. At what times of day does your child usually brush his/her teeth (or have them brushed for him/her)?

PLEASE TICK ALL THAT APPLY

- Before breakfast [1]
- After breakfast [2]
- Midday [3]
- Before the evening meal [4]
- After the evening meal [5]
- Before bed [6]
- Any other times (please tick and write in below) [7]

G
15 – 19
(MC = 5)

33. Have you or your child ever received any advice on the care of your child's teeth?

TICK ONE

- Yes, I have received advice [1] ── Go to Q34
- Yes, child has received advice [2] ── Go to Q34
- Yes, we have both received advice [3] ── Go to Q34
- No, neither of us have received advice [4] → Go to Q35

20

34. Who gave this advice?

PLEASE TICK ALL THAT APPLY

- Dentist [1]
- Doctor [2]
- Health Visitor [3]
- Dental Nurse [4]
- Dental Hygienist [5]
- Other (please tick and write in below) [6]

21 – 24
(MC = 4)

9

PLEASE DO NOT WRITE IN THIS COLUMN
G25

35. If the child has filled in questions 1 to 34 please tick the box.

[1]

So far we have asked questions about your child. We'd also like to know a little about you, his parents. Would you answer the following questions about both the parents of the child, if they live in the household. (Either parent may answer for both parents.) Please tick the boxes at the heads of the columns to show which parents live in the household. If only one parent lives in the household just answer for that parent.

	Mother	Father
36. Tick boxes to show which parents are in household.	[1]	[1]

26 – 27

37. Have you got some natural teeth or have you lost them all?	Mother	Father
Got some (all) natural teeth	[1]	[1]
Lost them all	[2]	[2]

28 – 29

38. In general do you go to the dentist for	Mother	Father
a regular check up	[1]	[1]
an occasional check up	[2]	[2]
or only when you are having trouble with your teeth?	[3]	[3]

30 – 31

39. How old are you?

PLEASE WRITE IN ON LINE ············→

32 – 35

40. At what age did you finish your full-time education?	Mother	Father
16 or under	[1]	[1]
17 or 18	[2]	[2]
Over 18	[3]	[3]

36 – 37

10

11

41. At the moment are you doing any paid work, either full or part time?

	Mother	Father
Yes full time	[1]	[1]
Yes part time	[2]	[2]
No	[3]	[3]

42. Could you tell us about the current job of the MOTHER of the child, or the last job she was in if she is no longer doing any paid work?

(If the mother of the child is not in the household please miss the question out and go to Q43.)

a) What is (or was) mother's job? (Please write in the job title)

b) What does (or did) mother actually do? (Please describe)

c) What does (or did) the firm or organization mother works (worked) for make or do?

d) Is mother (or was she) a manager or supervisor of any kind?

Yes manager [1]

Yes supervisor [2]

No neither [3]

12

43. Could you tell us about the current job of the FATHER of the child or the last job he was in if he is no longer doing any paid work. (If the father of the child is not in the household please miss this question out and go to Q44.)

a) What is (or was) father's job? (Please write in job title)

b) What does (or did) father actually do? (Please describe)

c) What does (or did) the firm or organization father works (worked) for make or do?

d) Is father (or was he) a manager or supervisor of any kind?

Yes manager [1]

Yes supervisor [2]

No neither [3]

44. Is there anything else you would like to say about dental health or dentistry?

Yes [1] → please write in below

No [2]

Thank you very much for your help.

Please do not forget to return this questionnaire in the reply paid envelope provided.

W2435B OPCS 12/82

S1189 CHILDRENS DENTAL HEALTH

DENTAL EXAMINATION

School Name _____

Child's Name _____

☐☐☐ Area Number

☐☐ School Number

☐☐☐ Child Number

(i) DATE OF BIRTH

Month Year

☐☐☐☐

(ii) AGE (YEARS)

☐☐

(iii) SEX

Male.............1
Female...........2

(iv) RACIAL ORIGIN

W Cauc...........1
Neg..............2
Pak/Ind..........3
Orien............4
Other (specify)..5
_____
Not Known........6

Dentist's name _____

☐☐ Dentist Number

Date of examination

Day Month

☐☐☐☐

IF NO EXAMINATION

Give reason why child not examined

---

1. TOOTH CONDITION

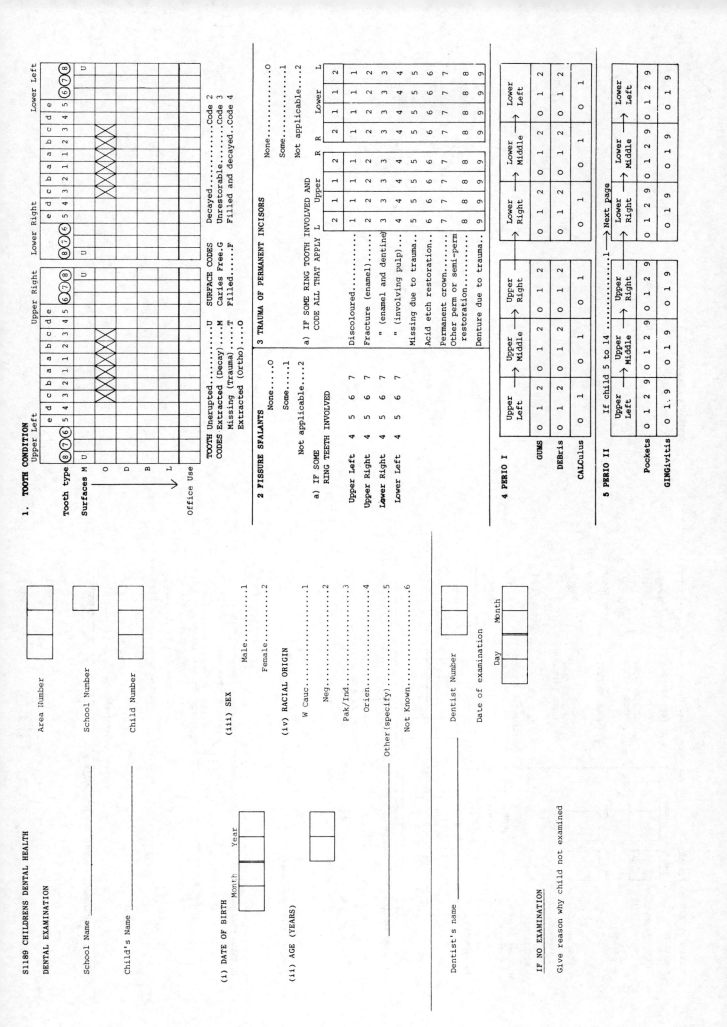

	Upper Right								Upper Left							
Tooth type	8	7	6	5	4	3	2	1	1	2	3	4	5	6	7	8
				e	d	c	b	a	a	b	c	d	e			
				5	4	3	2	1	1	2	3	4	5			

Surfaces M U
O
D
B
L

Office Use

	Lower Right								Lower Left							
	8	7	6	5	4	3	2	1	1	2	3	4	5	6	7	8
				e	d	c	b	a	a	b	c	d	e			
				5	4	3	2	1	1	2	3	4	5			

TOOTH   Unerupted................U
CODES   Extracted (Decay)....M
        Missing (Trauma).....T
        Extracted (Ortho)....O

SURFACE CODES
Caries Free..G
Filled.......F

Decayed..............Code 2
Unrestorable.........Code 3
Filled and decayed...Code 4

2 FISSURE SEALANTS

None.......0
Some.......1
Not applicable....2

a) IF SOME
   RING TEETH INVOLVED

Upper Left   4 5 6 7
Upper Right   4 5 6 7
Lower Right   4 5 6 7
Lower Left   4 5 6 7

3 TRAUMA OF PERMANENT INCISORS

None........0
Some........1
Not applicable..2

a) IF SOME RING TOOTH INVOLVED AND
   CODE ALL THAT APPLY

	Upper L		R R		Upper		Lower		L

	2	1	1	2	2	1	1	2
Discoloured...........	1	1	1	1	1	1	1	1
Fracture (enamel).....	2	2	2	2	2	2	2	2
" (enamel and dentine)	3	3	3	3	3	3	3	3
" (involving pulp)...	4	4	4	4	4	4	4	4
Missing due to trauma..	5	5	5	5	5	5	5	5
Acid etch restoration..	6	6	6	6	6	6	6	6
Permanent crown........	7	7	7	7	7	7	7	7
Other perm or semi-perm restoration............	8	8	8	8	8	8	8	8
Denture due to trauma..	9	9	9	9	9	9	9	9

4 PERIO I

	Upper Left	Upper Middle →	Upper Right	Lower Right →	Lower Middle →	Lower Left
GUMS	0 1 2	0 1 2	0 1 2	0 1 2	0 1 2	0 1 2
DEBris	0 1 2	0 1 2	0 1 2	0 1 2	0 1 2	0 1 2
CALCulus	0 1	0 1	0 1	0 1	0 1	0 1

5 PERIO II   If child 5 to 14 ....1 → Next page

	Upper Left	Upper Middle →	Upper Right	Lower Right →	Lower Middle →	Lower Left
Pockets	0 1 2 9	0 1 2 9	0 1 2 9	0 1 2 9	0 1 2 9	0 1 2 9
GINGivitis	0 1.9	0 1 9	0 1 9	0 1 9	0 1 9	0 1 9

147

PERMANENT INCISORS PRESENT   No permanent upper incisors present.....1 ⟶ 13

6 OVERJET

Upper Left   + / -   mms
Central Incisor

not assessed....9

Upper Right   + / -   mms
Central Incisor

not assessed......9

7 ROTATIONS

Any upper incisor rotated
30 degrees or more

| | None......0 | Some......1 |

8 a) INSTANDING

| | None.....0 | Some......1 |
(i) IF SOME RING
TEETH INVOLVED   Upper Left 1 2
                 Upper Right 1 2

b) EDGE TO EDGE

| | None.....0 | Some......1 |
(i) IF SOME RING
TEETH INVOLVED   Upper Left 1 2
                 Upper Right 1 2

9 TRAUMATIC OVERBITE

| | None.....0 | Some.....1 |

10 CROWDING

Upper Left	Upper Middle	Upper Right
0 1	0 1	0 1

Lower Right	Lower Middle	Lower Left
0 1	0 1	0 1

11 ORTHO APPLIANCE?   Has never worn appliance .... 1 ⟶ 12

Wearing appliance now 2   Has worn appliance 3
IF WEARING APPLIANCE   IF HAS WORN APPLIANCE
(a) Type of appliance   (b) Still wears it 4
                                      Finished with it 5

	Upper	Lower
None in this jaw	0	0
Removable	1	1
Fixed	2	2
Other (specify overleaf)	3	3

12 ORTHO TREATMENT NEED   Currently wears appliance ... 1 ⟶ 13

No treatment needed 0
Needs treatment 2   ⟶ IF NEEDS TREATMENT
                             a) Features requiring treatment
                                CODE ALL THAT APPLY
                                   Overjet........1
                                   Instanding incisor........2
                                   Rotated incisor.........3
                                   Gingival trauma........4
                                   Crowding........5
                             ⟵ Other (specify) 6

13 ASTERISK/COMMENTS RECORD DETAILS OVERLEAF

None.....0
Some.....1

148

W2435A OPCS 11/82

Printed in the UK for HMSO Dd 737848 C9 3/85